Fast Facts

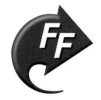

T027231

Fast Facts:
Cardiac
Arrhythmias

Second edition

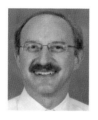

Gerry Kaye MBChB MD FRCP FRACP
Consultant Cardiologist and Associate Professor of
Cardiology
Department of Cardiology
Princess Alexandra Hospital
Woolloongabba, Brisbane, Australia

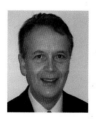

Steve Furniss MA MBBS FRCP
Consultant Cardiologist
East Sussex Hospitals NHS Trust
Eastbourne, East Sussex, UK

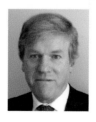

Robert Lemery MD FHRS FACC FRCP FESC
Clinical Cardiac Electrophysiology
Division of Cardiology
University of Ottawa Heart Institute
Ottawa, Ontario, Canada

Declaration of Independence
This book is as balanced and as pr
Ideas for improvement are always

D1421612

 HEALTH PRESS

Fast Facts: Cardiac Arrhythmias
First published 2010
Second edition May 2013; reprinted October 2015

Text © 2013 Gerry Kaye, Steve Furniss, Robert Lemery
© 2013 in this edition Health Press Limited
Health Press Limited, Elizabeth House, Queen Street, Abingdon,
Oxford OX14 3LN, UK
Tel: +44 (0)1235 523233
Fax: +44 (0)1235 523238

Book orders can be placed by telephone or via the website.
For regional distributors or to order via the website, please go to: fastfacts.com
For telephone orders, please call +44 (0)1752 202301 (UK, Europe and Asia–
Pacific), 1 800 247 6553 (USA, toll free) or +1 419 281 1802 (Americas).

Fast Facts is a trademark of Health Press Limited.

The publisher and the authors have made every effort to ensure the accuracy of this
book, but cannot accept responsibility for any errors or omissions.

For all drugs, please consult the product labeling approved in your country for
prescribing information.

A CIP record for this title is available from the British Library.

ISBN 978-1-908541-25-3

Kaye G (Gerry)
Fast Facts: Cardiac Arrhythmias/
Gerry Kaye, Steve Furniss, Robert Lemery

Medical illustrations by Dee McLean, London, UK.
Typesetting and page layout by Zed, Oxford, UK.
Printed by Charlesworth Press, Wakefield, UK.

Glossary and abbreviations

AF: atrial fibrillation

ARVC: arrhythmogenic right ventricular cardiomyopathy

ASA: acetylsalicylic acid (aspirin)

ATP: anti-tachycardia pacing

AV node: atrioventricular node

AVNRT: atrioventricular nodal re-entrant tachycardia (also described as junctional tachycardia)

AVRT: atrioventricular re-entrant tachycardia

bpm: beats per minute

CAD: coronary artery disease

Conduction: the speed at which cells propagate electrical wavefronts; different structures within the heart conduct at different rates (e.g. the His-Purkinje system conducts as rapidly as neural tissue [about 3 m/s], whereas conduction at the compact AV node is slower)

CRT: cardiac resynchronization therapy

DC: direct-current (cardioversion)

ECG: electrocardiogram

EP: electrophysiology

HCM: hypertrophic cardiomyopathy

ICD: implantable cardioverter defibrillator

INR: international normalized ratio

LAA: left atrial appendage

LQTS: long-QT syndrome

LV: left ventricular (function)

Macro or micro re-entrant arrhythmia: circuit that covers a large or small area of the myocardium, respectively

MI: myocardial infarction

NCT: narrow-(QRS)-complex tachycardia

PVI: pulmonary vein isolation

Refractoriness: as the rate of stimulation of a cardiac muscle cell (myocyte) increases, it will continue to contract until the external stimulus falls when the cell has not recovered its excitability from the previous stimulus; at this point the cell is refractory (i.e. it cannot respond to any stimulus)

RFA: radiofrequency ablation (also described as catheter ablation)

RVOT: right ventricular outflow tract

SA node: sinoatrial node

SVT: supraventricular tachycardia

VF: ventricular fibrillation

VKA: vitamin K antagonist

VT: ventricular tachycardia

WCT: Wide-(QRS)-complex tachycardia (also described as broad complex tachycardia)

WPW: Wolff–Parkinson–White (syndrome)

Introduction

Our understanding of cardiac arrhythmias has evolved so greatly over the past 20 years that clinical cardiac electrophysiology has been propelled into an important and effective subspecialty within medicine. Significantly, progress in interventional therapies has provided remarkable improvement in patient outcomes; for example, individuals who have been cured of their recurrent tachyarrhythmias or returned to living normal lives following implantation of a pacemaker or defibrillator.

This second edition of *Fast Facts: Cardiac Arrhythmias* continues its objective to provide a comprehensive easy-to-read review of the concepts of heart rhythm abnormality and the contemporary therapies available for patients with cardiac arrhythmias, with the ultimate aim of improving understanding, and thus patient care.

Cardiac arrhythmias are classified under 12-lead ECG patterns, with specific chapters relating to supraventricular arrhythmias, atrial flutter, atrial fibrillation, ventricular arrhythmias, and the rare but increasingly recognized inherited arrhythmias. Each well-illustrated chapter is divided into sections on how the patient presents and how they are best investigated and managed, using both pharmacological and non-pharmacological approaches. A final chapter covers pacemakers and implantable cardioverter defibrillators, the mainstay of therapy for patients with bradyarrhythmias, heart failure requiring biventricular pacing and ventricular tachyarrhythmias. MRI-compatible pacemakers are now used clinically.

Since the first edition of this book, the European Society of Cardiology has published new guidelines on the management of atrial fibrillation. The book has been revised to reflect these changes, as well as the latest thinking on catheter and surgical ablation and the most recent pharmacological updates, including the newer oral anticoagulants.

Warfarin, the commander in chief of anticoagulants for the past 50 years, may well be dethroned by a radical new approach to anticoagulation. Nonetheless, adherence will be crucial for patients taking once- or twice-daily non-warfarin oral anticoagulation.

Catheter ablation of all types of cardiac arrhythmias is performed worldwide, with excellent patient outcomes. New power sources and 3D non-fluoroscopic mapping systems continue to push the boundaries. Catheter ablation as first-line therapy has become standard in clinical practice, greatly alleviating symptoms in patients who for years have lived with recurrent, sometimes disabling and even fatal, cardiac arrhythmias.

We have thoroughly revised this succinct yet detailed handbook to keep abreast of the many changes that are taking place. We see *Fast Facts: Cardiac Arrhythmias* as a must-read resource for all general practitioners, nurses, medical students, technicians and cardiologists in training looking for a concise up-to-date overview of this dynamic field of modern cardiology.

Conduction within the heart

Normal conduction

Cardiac cells have a unique ability to depolarize rhythmically. Normally, depolarization within the heart occurs in one direction from the top downwards. The fibrous ring that supports the mitral and tricuspid valves is an electrical insulator, so depolarization can only travel from the atria to the ventricles via the specialized conducting tissues, unless an abnormal electrically active connection, known as an accessory pathway, is present (see Chapter 2). The normal conduction pathway within the heart is described below (Figure 1.1).

Atrial depolarization. Conduction originates with self-excitation of the sinoatrial (SA) node, which lies at the junction of the superior vena cava with the upper part of the right atrium. The SA node acts as the heart's pacemaker. A depolarization wavefront spreads down from the SA node to the base of the right atrium and simultaneously spreads to the left atrium over specialized conductive tissue known as Bachmann's bundle. The complete depolarization of the atria gives rise to the P wave on the surface electrocardiogram (ECG; see Figure 1.1). A normal P wave is less than 200 ms wide and smaller than 1 mV in amplitude. It has a low amplitude because the mass of the atria is considerably smaller than that of the ventricles. The P wave is wide because most of the depolarization of the atria occurs by relatively slow cell-to-cell conduction.

Atrioventricular node depolarization. The depolarization wavefront is then directed to the compact atrioventricular (AV) node, which bridges the atria and ventricles near the center of the heart. Conduction through the AV node is slowed in the upper part of the node. This delay allows mechanical contraction of the atria, which is much slower than the electrical activation, to complete before the ventricles contract, and gives rise to the PR interval on the surface ECG (less than 200 ms).

Septal depolarization. Once through the AV node, the wavefront travels through the septum and reaches the specialized His-Purkinje system.

(a)

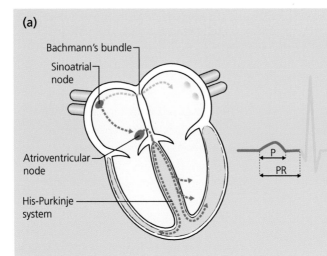

Figure 1.1 Normal conduction pathway within the heart, with corresponding surface ECG. (a) The cardiac impulse arises from the sinoatrial node and depolarizes the atria by cell-to-cell conduction and via Bachmann's bundle, giving rise to the P wave on the ECG. The impulse is slowed through the atrioventricular node, which corresponds to the PR interval on the ECG. The impulse is then conducted rapidly to the His-Purkinje system and bundle branches. (b) The ventricles are depolarized via the His-Purkinje system, giving rise to the narrow QRS complex on the ECG. (c) Electrical recovery of the ventricles corresponds to the T wave. The QT interval is measured from the onset of the QRS complex to a point where the down stroke of the T wave crosses the baseline; the faster the heart beat the shorter the QT interval.

The His tissue conducts rapidly and, after splitting to follow the left and right bundle branches, the wavefront depolarizes the ventricles.

Ventricular depolarization and systole. The mass of ventricular tissue far outweighs that of the atria. Hence, the amplitude of electrical depolarization of the ventricles (represented by the surface QRS complex) is much greater than that in the atria. The QRS width is also relatively narrow because of the specialized conducting tissues of the His-Purkinje system, which includes the bundle branches of the ventricles.

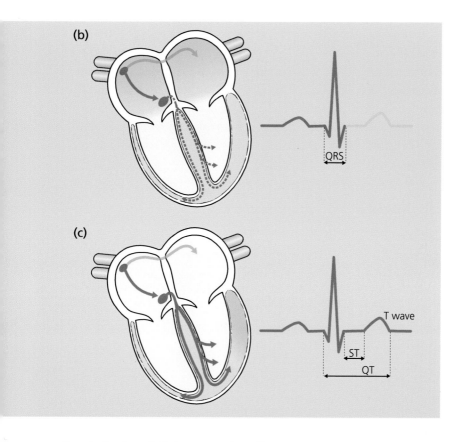

(b)

QRS

(c)

T wave

ST

QT

Depolarization of all the ventricular cells causes myocardial contraction and ventricular systole. The isoelectric ST segment and T wave correspond with electrical recovery of the ventricles.

Ventricular repolarization and diastole. After contracting, the heart muscle relaxes and the membrane potential recovers, appearing as the T wave on the ECG. When the heart has completely repolarized, the heart muscle is fully relaxed and there is no electrical activity until the SA node triggers the start of the next beat.

Electrical properties of the atrioventricular node

The conduction properties of the AV node are unique. As discussed earlier, the AV node slows conduction before the impulse reaches the His-Purkinje fibers and ventricles. Under normal circumstances, the AV node transmits every beat from the atria to the ventricles (1:1), usually up to 150–180 beats per minute (bpm). Thereafter, the AV node will begin to block conduction. This takes the form of progressive lengthening of the PR interval until a single beat is blocked, known as the Wenckebach phenomenon, and is a normal feature of AV nodal conduction at high heart rates (Figure 1.2). At even higher heart rates, the frequency of this block increases (higher grade AV block) such that every second or third beat no longer gets through the AV node.

This slowing phenomenon of AV nodal tissue is known as decremental conduction and is characteristic of the AV node (accessory pathways very

(a)

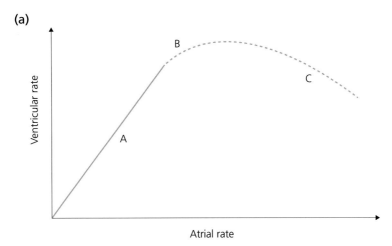

(b)

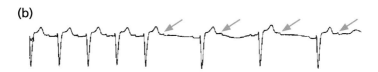

Figure 1.2 (a) Decremental conduction of the atrioventricular (AV) node. A, as the atrial rate increases the ventricular rate increases in a linear fashion. B, as the atrial rate increases further the ventricular rate beings to 'slow', the PR interval increases and occasional atrial beats fail to conduct to the ventricles (Wenckebach phenomenon). C, at some point (which is age related), more atrial beats are blocked and the level of ventricular block increases. (b) Surface ECG showing sinus rhythm followed by 2:1 AV nodal block. The arrows show the second P wave, which is not conducted to the ventricles. The QRS is narrow.

rarely demonstrate decrementation). Decremental conduction of the AV node is age related. The heart rate required to produce Wenckebach block decreases with age: for example, at 20–40 years Wenckebach block occurs at 160–180 bpm, whereas over 70 years of age it occurs at approximately 120 bpm. Despite this relative slowing effect, it is still possible to maintain very rapid heart rates during tachycardia, emphasizing how complex conduction within the heart can be. Wenckebach phenomenon is common at night; Holter monitoring (see page 42) often reveals frequent pauses during sleep in otherwise healthy young people. This type of AV block usually does not require treatment. Some antiarrhythmic drugs also slow AV nodal conduction and may cause Wenckebach phenomenon.

Influence of the autonomic nervous system

Although the heart muscle has intrinsic rhythmicity, an individual's heart rate is influenced by outside factors and can vary widely during the day, reflecting the relative balance between the sympathetic and parasympathetic nervous systems. For example, in the 'flight or fright' response to danger, the sympathetic system activates the adrenal glands and releases epinephrine (adrenaline) into the circulation. This stimulates cardiac beta-adrenoreceptors, generally increasing cardiac conduction, heart rate and the force of contraction. Conversely, the parasympathetic system, via the vagus nerve, has a dampening effect, reducing the heart rate and force of contraction. Intracardiac conduction is slowed and in certain patients AV nodal conduction can be slowed significantly. Maneuvers that provoke a vagal response, such as carotid sinus massage or vomiting, may terminate arrhythmias that use the AV node as part of their mechanism (e.g. many supraventricular tachycardias, SVTs). Profound vagal activation usually produces a specific sequence of prodromal symptoms: for 1–2 minutes patients complain of feeling light-headed and nauseous, followed by sweating and worsening nausea; they may ultimately lose consciousness as a result of severe bradycardias or hypotension. Other factors such as thyroid hormones and pregnancy also affect heart rate.

Carotid sinus massage. The carotid sinus is a heavily innervated structure that lies in the common carotid artery at the level of the cricoid cartilage. Gentle but steady massage of this sinus induces a neural reflex, the efferent arm of which is the vagus nerve to the heart. This produces a degree of sinus slowing but also a slowing in AV nodal conduction, to the point of producing AV block in some patients. This is a useful means of terminating some arrhythmias (usually SVTs) and may also show the underlying nature of an arrhythmia. For example, increasing AV block in atrial flutter 'brings out' the flutter P waves and establishes the diagnosis.

Key points – conduction within the heart

- Cardiac cells have the unique ability to depolarize rhythmically; depolarization normally occurs in one direction from the top down, from atria to ventricles.
- The fibrous atrioventricular (AV) ring, which supports the mitral and tricuspid valves, behaves as an electrical insulator: conduction to the ventricles occurs only over the AV node unless there is an abnormal or aberrant connection.
- The AV node has a decremental slowing effect on conduction.
- Autonomic effects on the heart (sympathetic and parasympathetic stimuli) can significantly influence cardiac conduction.

2 Classification and mechanisms of arrhythmias

A simple classification of arrhythmias is based on the site at which the primary anatomic abnormality arises (Table 2.1). The most common arrhythmias are discussed in greater detail in subsequent chapters.

Mechanisms of arrhythmia

Generally, arrhythmias can be divided into two broad mechanisms:
- a disorder of impulse formation – abnormal automaticity or triggered activity
- a disorder of impulse conduction – re-entry.

The major mechanism in humans is re-entry, which is detailed in the following sections along with a brief overview of other mechanisms.

Disorders of impulse formation are uncommon. Disorders in this category are characterized by an inappropriate discharge rate from the sinoatrial (SA) node or an ectopic pacemaker. There are two types: abnormal automaticity and triggered activity.

Abnormal automaticity. Automaticity is the property of a myocyte to initiate an impulse spontaneously without prior stimulation. Slow atrial,

---

TABLE 2.1

Classification of arrhythmias by anatomic site

- Sinus node re-entry
- Supraventricular tachycardia (SVT)
  - atrioventricular re-entrant tachycardia (AVRT)
  - atrioventricular nodal re-entrant tachycardia (AVNRT) (also termed junctional re-entrant tachycardia; JRT)

- Atrial tachycardia
  - automatic
  - focal
  - multifocal
- Atrial flutter
- Atrial fibrillation
- Ventricular tachycardia
- Ventricular fibrillation

junctional and ventricular escape rhythms are automatic in nature. Atrial tachycardias linked to digitalis overdose are also thought to be of this type. It is thought the commonest 'arrhythmias' – ventricular and atrial ectopics – also arise from this mechanism.

Triggered activity is when pacemaker activity arises as a consequence of a preceding impulse or series of impulses. These are thought to account for more unusual arrhythmias associated with, for example, the long-QT syndrome (see Chapter 10), either congenital or acquired (usually drug-induced or with coronary ischemia). Polymorphic ventricular tachycardias are thought to be of this type (see Chapter 9).

Disorders of impulse conduction (re-entry) form the basis of almost all major arrhythmias in humans, and require two pathological features:

- a substrate – an abnormal pathway or connection that allows a depolarizing wavefront to re-enter an area that it would not normally enter; often the wavefront circulates around a fixed, usually anatomic, obstacle (e.g. a scar)
- a trigger – a feature that initiates the arrhythmia: the most common form is an atrial or ventricular ectopic beat.

Accessory pathways. The best-described mechanism of re-entry is that due to an accessory pathway – an abnormal connection between the atria and ventricle that bypasses the specialized conducting tissues of the atrioventricular (AV) node and His-Purkinje system. These accessory pathways (also known as bypass tracts) are usually anatomically separate from the specialized conducting tissue (Figure 2.1).

Narrow versus wide (broad) QRS complexes

In addition to the anatomically based classification described above, electrophysiologists use a 'narrow versus wide QRS' classification for arrhythmias, which allows the prediction of outcome and prognosis.

Narrow-complex tachycardias (NCTs) during an arrhythmia mean that depolarization of the ventricles occurs via the specialized system of the AV node and the His-Purkinje system. This usually occurs during SVT and nearly always signifies a non-life-threatening arrhythmia. An NCT implies the presence of some sort of aberrant

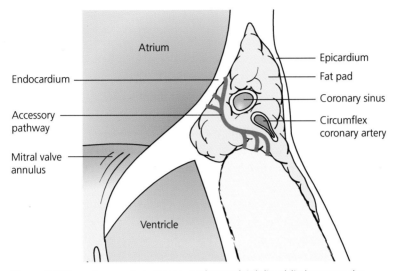

Figure 2.1 The microscopic accessory pathways (pink lines) lie between the atrial and ventricular myocardium within the epicardial fat pads.

electrical pathway (e.g. an accessory pathway or slow/fast pathways) as the underlying mechanism or, less frequently, an atrial tachycardia.

Wide-complex tachycardias (WCTs) have three possible causes:
- a problem with the specialized conducting tissue
- bypassing of the specialized conducting tissue
- impulses that arise in the ventricles outside the specialized conducting tissue.

Although WCTs can occur during SVT, they are uncommon. *For all practical purposes a WCT should be considered ventricular in origin until proven otherwise and treated accordingly.* Ventricular tachycardia (VT) nearly always carries a poor prognosis and needs urgent and specialized treatment (see Chapter 9). Inappropriate drug management of a WCT can be dangerous or even fatal.

Sinus node re-entry tachycardia

This is a rare and unusual arrhythmia whereby the sinus node is driven by a micro-re-entrant circuit arising within the node. The surface ECG looks like an inappropriate and persistent sinus tachycardia. Other causes such as thyrotoxicosis and pregnancy need to be excluded.

Supraventricular tachycardia

SVT is a general term encompassing a number of arrhythmias that arise within the atria or AV node and produce a regular rapid heart rate. Most have narrow QRS complexes on the surface ECG, demonstrating that depolarization of the ventricles occurs over the His-Purkinje system.

Wolff–Parkinson–White (WPW) syndrome. The best-described re-entrant circuit occurs in WPW syndrome. Although it affects only about 0.01% of the population, WPW syndrome accounts for about 20% of SVTs. In these patients, an accessory pathway (sometimes referred to as a bundle of Kent) exists in addition to the normal conduction pathway; occasionally, more than one pathway occurs in the same patient. The characteristics of these pathways are highlighted in Table 2.2.

During sinus rhythm the impulse spreads from the SA node in its usual manner and depolarizes both atria. Conduction is slowed through the AV node as normal, but it is not slowed through the accessory pathway. The impulse from the atria is therefore partly conducted to the ventricles via this route rather than only through the AV node and His-Purkinje system. This allows part of the ventricle to depolarize before it would otherwise do so (overt pre-excitation), resulting in a diagnostic abnormality on the surface ECG – fusion of the P wave with the initial part of the QRS complex, demonstrating depolarization from both normal AV node conduction and through the accessory pathway (Figure 2.2). This slurring of the upstroke of the initial part of the QRS deflection, called a delta wave, causes the QRS to be wider than normal. It can sometimes be confused with the appearance of bundle branch block, which also causes a broadening of the QRS because of abnormal depolarization of the ventricles. The delta wave vector can be used to determine the position of the accessory pathways.

Sustained arrhythmia in the WPW syndrome requires both an accessory pathway (the substrate) and a trigger, which is almost always an ectopic beat, either atrial or ventricular. These ectopic beats need to be critically timed in order to initiate the arrhythmia (Figure 2.3). The fact that people with accessory pathways have arrhythmias only now and again emphasizes the relative infrequency at which an ectopic beat falls at a critical time to allow the arrhythmia to start.

A critically timed atrial or ventricular ectopic beat during the tachycardia can also terminate an arrhythmia if the ectopic depolarizes the

TABLE 2.2

Characteristics of accessory pathways in WPW syndrome

- Situated anywhere on the AV ring connecting the atria to the ventricles
- Usually pass from the atrial myocardium through the epicardial fat into the ventricular myocardium (see Figure 2.1)
- Microscopic; rarely found postmortem
- Electrical characteristics similar to the His-Purkinje system – rapid conduction and no slowing with increasing heart rate (unlike AV nodal tissue)
- Conduct in a 1:1 fashion at increasing heart rates (incremental conduction); can conduct very rapidly
- Can conduct from the atria to the ventricles (antegrade conduction) as well as from the ventricles to the atria (retrograde conduction)

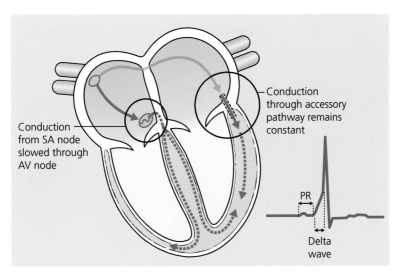

Figure 2.2 Wolff–Parkinson–White syndrome. Conduction is slowed through the AV node as normal but it is not slowed through the accessory pathway, allowing part of the ventricle to depolarize early (overt pre-excitation). The corresponding ECG shows a short PR interval (as the AV node is bypassed), fusion of the (normal) P wave with the initial part of the QRS complex, an upsloping of the initial QRS deflection (a delta wave), creating a wide QRS complex, and an abnormal T wave that is usually inverted or biphasic.

part of the heart that lies in front of the circulating wavefront, creating an area of refractoriness as the tachycardia wavefront arrives.

Antegrade and retrograde conduction. In the WPW syndrome, the accessory pathway is usually capable of both antegrade (atrium to ventricle) and retrograde (ventricle to atrium) conduction. During sinus rhythm, antegrade conduction causes the surface ECG to be abnormal as described above, indicating the presence of the accessory pathway. This appearance on the surface ECG (short PR interval and a delta wave) is known as overt pre-excitation (see Figure 2.2).

Orthodromic tachycardia occurs in 95% of patients with WPW, with the arrhythmia circuitry exhibiting antegrade conduction through the AV node and His-Purkinje system and retrograde conduction over the accessory pathway (see Figure 2.3). During SVT, the QRS complexes are narrow, as ventricular depolarization occurs normally via the His-Purkinje system.

Antidromic tachycardia occurs in fewer than 5% of cases. The circuit is reversed such that antegrade conduction occurs over the pathway and

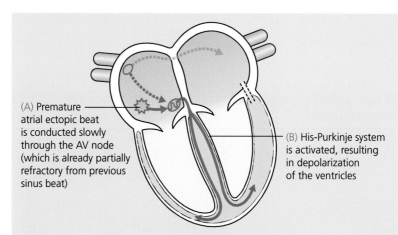

(A) Premature atrial ectopic beat is conducted slowly through the AV node (which is already partially refractory from previous sinus beat)

(B) His-Purkinje system is activated, resulting in depolarization of the ventricles

Figure 2.3 Sustained arrhythmia (orthodromic tachycardia) in Wolff–Parkinson–White syndrome, showing antegrade conduction (atrium to ventricle) over the AV node and His-Purkinje system, followed by retrograde conduction (ventricle to atrium) over the accessory pathway. The corresponding ECG shows narrow QRS complexes as the ventricles are depolarized over the fast conducting tissue of the His-Purkinje system.

returns to the atria via the His-Purkinje system. The ventricles are fully pre-excited and the QRS complexes are therefore wide, often very wide (Figure 2.4). This tachycardia is often misdiagnosed (not unreasonably) as ventricular in origin.

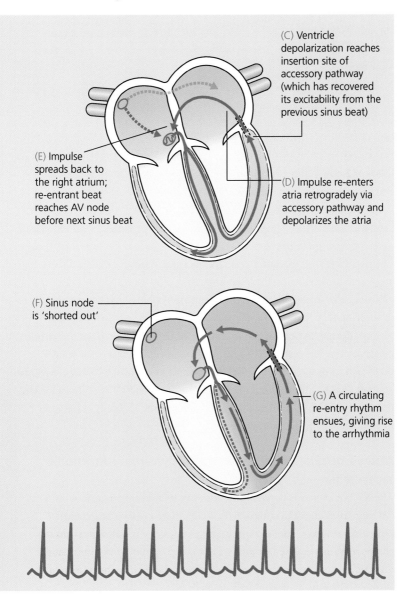

(C) Ventricle depolarization reaches insertion site of accessory pathway (which has recovered its excitability from the previous sinus beat)

(E) Impulse spreads back to the right atrium; re-entrant beat reaches AV node before next sinus beat

(D) Impulse re-enters atria retrogradely via accessory pathway and depolarizes the atria

(F) Sinus node is 'shorted out'

(G) A circulating re-entry rhythm ensues, giving rise to the arrhythmia

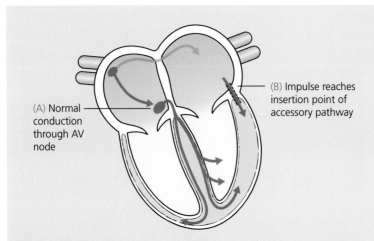

(A) Normal conduction through AV node

(B) Impulse reaches insertion point of accessory pathway

Figure 2.4 Antidromic tachycardia in Wolff–Parkinson–White syndrome, showing antegrade conduction (atrium to ventricle) over the accessory pathway and retrograde conduction (ventricle to atrium) via the His-Purkinje system. The corresponding ECG shows wide QRS complexes as the ventricles are not depolarized over the His-Purkinje system but via the accessory pathway and then through the ventricular myocardium.

Concealed accessory pathways. Electrophysiology has shown that in some patients with SVTs, the accessory pathway is capable of only retrograde conduction, so pre-excitation of the ventricles from the atrium never occurs. The resting ECG is therefore normal. These concealed pathways form the substrate for a significant number of SVTs and they are another cause of narrow-complex tachycardia. The SVT mechanism is the same as for SVTs in pre-excitation syndromes (see Figure 2.2) but only orthodromic tachycardias are possible.

Atrioventricular nodal re-entrant tachycardia / Junctional tachycardia

The AV nodal area is complex. In addition to a discrete region within the AV ring, known as the compact AV node, there are two anatomically separate pathways – the slow and fast pathways – which input into the compact AV node. The fast pathway conducts rapidly but 'wears out' quickly (a short refractory period), whereas the slow pathway conducts slowly and recovers more slowly as well.

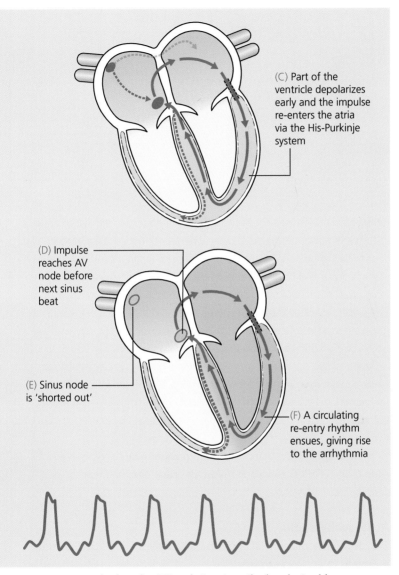

(C) Part of the ventricle depolarizes early and the impulse re-enters the atria via the His-Purkinje system

(D) Impulse reaches AV node before next sinus beat

(E) Sinus node is 'shorted out'

(F) A circulating re-entry rhythm ensues, giving rise to the arrhythmia

During sinus rhythm the AV node is primarily depolarized by an impulse running over the fast pathway, rendering it refractory to the impulse from the slow pathway. However, a critically timed ectopic can lead to an atrioventricular nodal re-entrant tachycardia (AVNRT), also known as junctional re-entrant tachycardia, which has a narrow QRS complex on the surface ECG (Figure 2.5).

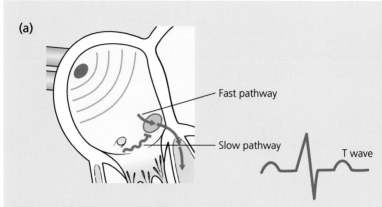

(a)

Fast pathway

Slow pathway

T wave

Figure 2.5 (a) A sinus beat depolarizes the AV node over the fast pathway. (b) If a premature atrial ectopic arises it may reach the AV node when the fast pathway is refractory, in which case the impulse 'jumps' to the slow pathway, conducting through the AV node antegradely and then through the His-Purkinje system. (c) However, by the time the atrial ectopic has passed to the AV node the fast pathway has recovered its excitability and the impulse can be conducted retrogradely over the fast pathway back to the atrium (atrial echo beat). If this retrograde atrial beat reaches the atrial insertion of the slow pathway when it has recovered, (d) a re-entrant circuit will be established between the slow and fast pathways giving rise to an atrioventricular re-entrant tachycardia (AVNRT) with a narrow-QRS-complex tachycardia.

Within AVNRT there are occasional unusual forms – types B and C – but most AVNRTs (about 95%) are the more common type A, as described in Figure 2.5.

Atrial tachycardia

The mechanism of an atrial tachycardia is either an automatic focus or a re-entrant rhythm occurring within a small area of the atrial myocardium. An automatic focus usually arises in a discrete part of the atrium and is triggered by autonomic stimuli (usually epinephrine [adrenaline]), for example with exercise. Such arrhythmias are hard to initiate during electrophysiological (EP) studies and often are initiated only with isoprenaline (isoproterenol). A focal atrial tachycardia has a micro re-entrant mechanism that is localized to a small area of the atrium;

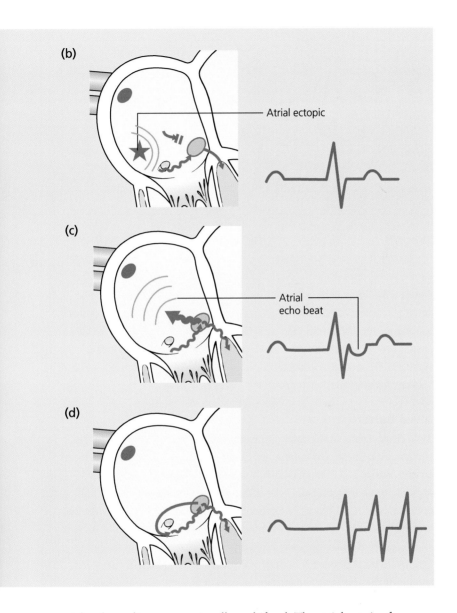

atrial tachycardias are occasionally multifocal. The atrial rate is often 150–250 bpm. The P wave morphology on the surface ECG often gives a clue as to the origin of the arrhythmia. If, as is more usual, the abnormal area is localized, it can be treated by focal ablation, which is usually successful (Figure 2.6).

23

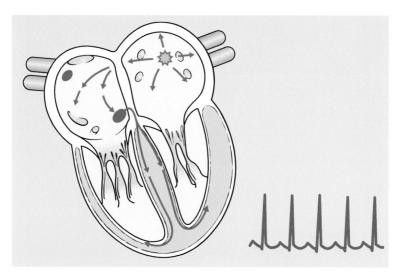

Figure 2.6 A focus in the atria can cause an atrial tachycardia. These can be automatic, epinephrine (adrenaline)-sensitive or re-entrant, arising from either a localized area anywhere in the atrial tissue (micro re-entrant) or from a larger area of tissue (macro re-entrant; see Glossary, page 4). The corresponding surface ECG shows atrial tachycardia, with the P waves superimposed on the T waves, making interpretation of the P wave vector difficult.

Atrial flutter

Typical, or classic, atrial flutter is a re-entrant rhythm that usually rotates counterclockwise or, less commonly, clockwise within the body of the right atrium (Figure 2.7). The atrial rate is usually 300 bpm. The ventricular response is often regular and related directly to the atrial rate depending on the degree of AV block. The commonest form is 2:1 AV block where the ventricular rate is regular at 150 bpm. Higher rates of block, 3:1 or 4:1, are also seen, often when antiarrhythmic drugs are used to control the flutter.

The circuit depends on an area of critical slow conduction that most commonly lies between the inferior vena cava and the tricuspid valve, known as the right atrial or, more precisely, the cavotricuspid isthmus. The P waves in typical atrial flutter usually have a saw-tooth appearance (flutter waves) in the 12-lead ECG (see Figure 2.7).

Atypical atrial flutter follows a different re-entry pathway that is not dependent on the cavotricuspid isthmus. It may occur after cardiac surgery

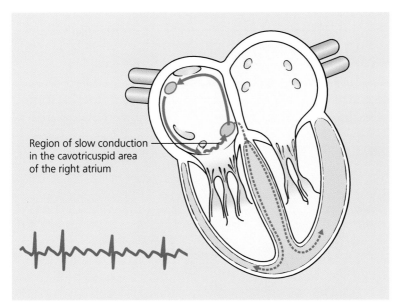

Region of slow conduction in the cavotricuspid area of the right atrium

Figure 2.7 Mechanism of typical atrial flutter. The abnormal circuit rotates, usually counterclockwise, within the atria and is maintained by an abnormal area of slow conduction known as the cavotricuspid isthmus. The surface ECG of typical atrial flutter shows the characteristic saw-tooth pattern of P waves.

(e.g. closure of an atrial septal defect) or left atrial flutter may occur after ablation for atrial fibrillation (AF). Atypical flutter can occur many years after surgery (e.g. in patients who have had previous surgery to correct a congenital defect), with the circuit rotating around the surgical scar.

Atrial fibrillation

AF is now thought to be related to a complex re-entry mechanism. Several types of AF are clinically recognized:

- paroxysmal – usually recurrent but lasting fewer than 7 days and self-terminating
- persistent – lasting longer than 7 days and requiring intervention for termination
- long-standing persistent – continuous AF that lasts for 1 year or more while a rhythm control strategy is pursued
- permanent – decision is made by the cardiologist not to attempt termination.

25

Studies of paroxysmal AF have revealed foci of atrial triggers, in general arising within the pulmonary veins at their junction with the left atrium (Figure 2.8). These foci are thought to be due to thin slivers of atrial tissue lying within the veins, with localized autonomic ganglia releasing neurotransmitters. The vein may contain many of these abnormal fibers, which fire repetitively and give rise to frequent ectopics that depolarize

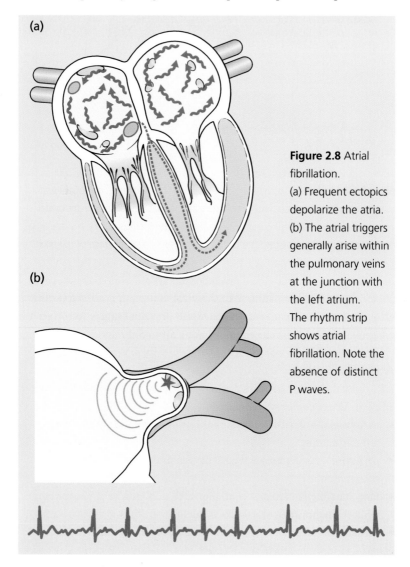

(a)

(b)

Figure 2.8 Atrial fibrillation.
(a) Frequent ectopics depolarize the atria.
(b) The atrial triggers generally arise within the pulmonary veins at the junction with the left atrium.
The rhythm strip shows atrial fibrillation. Note the absence of distinct P waves.

the atria. It is believed that over time the frequency increases to a degree where the rhythm breaks down into multiple small re-entrant wavelets, giving rise to recurrent paroxysmal AF and, in some patients, persistent AF. Ultimately, both the anatomy and electrical stability of the atria are altered and combine to make the development of AF more likely. This form of paroxysmal AF is occasionally referred to as 'focal AF'.

In persistent, long-standing persistent and permanent AF, additional changes occur within the atria over time: increased fibrosis, and changes in atrial refractoriness and conduction. These changes promote areas of re-entry within the body of the left atrium that maintain the AF.

In contrast to typical atrial flutter, AF is most often a left atrial disorder (occasionally AF drivers are also right-sided).

Ventricular tachycardia

The most common type of ventricular tachycardia (VT) is related to ischemic heart disease or cardiomyopathic processes. Less commonly, and usually in younger patients, VT arises in a structurally normal heart.

During normal conduction the depolarizing wavefront arrives at a constant speed within the ventricular myocardium. Recovery occurs at a constant speed in the opposite direction to depolarization (see Chapter 1). During a myocardial infarction, although there may be areas of tissue death that are unable to depolarize, there are also coexisting areas of ischemia. Conduction and recovery are variably slow in these ischemic areas (the substrate) and if an impulse is slowed sufficiently it may re-enter a nearby area that has recovered conduction and that may now allow a re-entrant circuit to occur (Figure 2.9). Ventricular ectopics are often the trigger.

Sometimes the VT circuit covers a relatively large area and may have complex re-entry circuits. These are often deep within the myocardium and occur over a relatively large area, which is why ablation is often difficult and less successful than if the abnormal substrate area is microscopic (as in SVTs).

Ventricular fibrillation

Ventricular fibrillation (VF) is now thought to have a re-entrant basis. It most commonly occurs during (or after) myocardial infarction or ischemia; less often it is related to electrolyte disturbance or drug therapy.

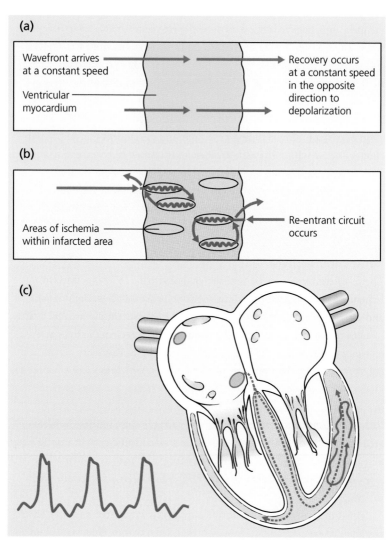

Figure 2.9 (a) In normal ventricular myocardium, depolarization and electrical recovery are uniform. (b) Following a myocardial infarction or ischemia, areas of damaged but viable tissue depolarize and recover more slowly than surrounding tissues. These areas allow impulses to re-enter locally thereby establishing a tachycardia, which may arise within a relatively small area of the ventricle but (c) spreads out to involve the remainder of the ventricular myocardium, giving rise to ventricular tachycardia. The surface ECG shows very wide (broad) QRS complexes.

VF has been described in 'normal' hearts and is often related to an early-cycle ventricular ectopic falling within the vulnerable period of ventricular recovery. Ablation of these ectopics has been shown to prevent recurrent fibrillation. It is thought that these ectopics allow localized re-entry.

Key points – classification and mechanisms of arrhythmias

- Re-entry is the most frequent mechanism for arrhythmias.
- The substrate for an arrhythmia is an abnormal electrical pathway or a region of scarred myocardium. The trigger is an atrial or ventricular ectopic beat.
- Narrow-QRS-complex arrhythmias signify depolarization of the ventricle over the usual His-Purkinje system.
- Most supraventricular tachycardias have narrow QRS complexes.
- Wide (broad)-complex tachycardias need further investigation, and patients should be referred for urgent assessment. *They should be considered ventricular in origin until proven otherwise.*

Key references

Akhtar M, Shenasa M, Jazayeri M et al. Wide QRS complex tachycardia: reappraisal of a common clinical problem. *Ann Intern Med* 1988;109: 905–12.

De Bacquer D, De Backer G, Kornitzer M. Prevalences of ECG findings in large population based samples of men and women. *Heart* 2000;84:625–33.

Goudevenos JA, Katsouras CS, Graekas G et al. Ventricular pre-excitation in the general population: a study on the mode of presentation and clinical course. *Heart* 2000;83:29–34.

Libby P, Bonow RO, Zipes DP, Mann DL, eds. *Braunwald's Heart Disease: A Textbook of Cardiovascular Medicine*, 8th edn. Saunders, 2007.

Rowlands DJ. Understanding the Electrocardiogram: *The Normal ECG Pt. 1: A New Approach*. Churchill Livingstone, 1981.

Surawicz B, Knilans TK, eds. *Chou's Electrocardiography in Clinical Practice: Adult and Pediatric*, 6th edn. Philadelphia: Saunders, 2008.

Wellens HJ, Bär FW, Lie KI. The value of the electrocardiogram in the differential diagnosis of a tachycardia with a widened QRS complex. *Am J Med* 1978;64:27–33.

Patients with cardiac arrhythmias can present with any of the following symptoms:

- palpitations – the baseline symptom for all arrhythmias
- breathlessness/fatigue
- falls/blackouts (syncope – complete loss of consciousness – and pre-syncope, which is the sensation patients describe of a near blackout without actually being aware of blacking out)
- chest pains (although it is relatively unusual to present solely with chest pains)
- resuscitated sudden death – the patient is resuscitated from a cardiac arrest, usually as a result of ventricular fibrillation (VF) or tachycardia (VT) out of hospital
- no cardiac symptoms at all (e.g. with atrial fibrillation [AF] after a stroke, or as a finding at screening).

There are often few or no physical signs, and although cardiovascular examination may be normal, this does not rule out a cardiac cause. Patients with chest pain, rhythm disturbance or murmurs need further investigation.

Palpitations

Palpitations are common in patients with any cardiac arrhythmia. When interviewing a patient with palpitations it is important to determine whether the palpitations represent abnormal awareness of a normal heart beat or an actual cardiac rhythm disturbance (i.e. normal awareness of an abnormal beat). Try to get the patient to be as clear as possible in their description, and ask them to tap out what they feel their heart is actually doing. Table 3.1 highlights some of the key questions to ask your patient, which will help with the diagnosis.

Palpitation is the baseline symptom for all arrhythmias but there are few specific symptoms that differentiate one rhythm from another. The occurrence of other symptoms depends on factors such as the patient's premorbid fitness level and the presence or absence of underlying cardiac disease. For example, a 20-year-old with atrial arrhythmia or

TABLE 3.1

Key questions to ask the patient at first presentation

- Is your heart beating fast or just strongly?
- Is it regular or irregular ('all over the place')?
- Does it start suddenly or gradually speed up?
- Does it stop suddenly or gradually ease off?
- How long does it last for?
- Is it starting and stopping or is it there all the time?
- How does it make you feel?
- Do you get any warning symptoms?
- Can you do anything to stop it?*
- What brings it on?
- Are you going to the toilet more frequently to pass urine?†

*Patients commonly attempt to terminate arrhythmias by breath holding.
†Polyuria is an unusual symptom; although rare, it nearly always occurs in a supraventricular tachycardia or atrial fibrillation.

supraventricular tachycardia (SVT) may not have many symptoms other than palpitations, whereas a 60-year-old with mitral stenosis or regurgitation may have severe symptoms such as shortness of breath or even pulmonary edema. Sometimes patients will notice that their palpitations feel irregular, suggesting AF, but this is not a consistent or reliable observation and it can be difficult to determine whether or not the heart is regular at fast rates.

Increased awareness of a normal heart beat may be more apparent in those who have sinus rhythm only. Issues to look for include:
- a family history of cardiac disease
- a previous cardiac history
- a previous history of neurotic symptoms.

Individuals who have had a previous cardiac abnormality or who have a family history of cardiac disease may have increased awareness of their own heart beat. For example, following a successful ablation it is common for patients to become aware of ectopics, the trigger beats that previously started a sustained arrhythmia. This can be mitigated by warning your patient that they are likely to be more aware of their heart beat for several months after an ablation procedure.

Cardiac rhythm disturbance

The normal heart beat is not entirely regular; the sinus node is under autonomic control and is influenced by breathing and exercise (see Chapter 1). In the young, marked variation in the heart rate with breathing may occur; this is normal and is termed sinus arrhythmia and is sometimes noticed by patients who take their own pulse frequently.

Ectopics arise through firing of ventricular or atrial foci and the symptoms often have three components:
- 'the early beat' – the ectopic itself
- 'the gap' – the postectopic pause (often described as the heart missing a beat, stopping or skipping)
- 'the thump' – postectopic potentiation.

Although the sensation is abnormal, some patients do not notice the ectopic itself because of the reduced filling time and reduced stroke volume. Usually, the more frequent the ectopics (e.g. 5% of the day), the more likely the patient is to notice. Conversely, some patients who have one or two ectopics per day can feel every one of them.

Symptomatic atrial ectopy is rare but salvos of atrial ectopy can occur (sometimes as a prodrome to the onset of AF) and may cause symptoms. Symptoms are more common with ventricular ectopics, which are associated with a greater disturbance to hemodynamic function. Symptoms are related to uncoordinated ventricular contraction, causing abnormal movement of the heart within the chest, or due to retrograde atrial activation and contraction of the atria against closed atrioventricular (AV) valves. Patients often use terms such as 'fullness', 'tightening' or 'swelling' in the upper chest or neck and may describe pressure in the neck due to regurgitation of blood into the jugular veins.

Typically, benign ectopics arise after exercise (when the sinus node slows down rapidly but the catecholamines produced during exercise are still circulating and cause firing of cells), during rest when the patient is lying on their left side (due to the mechanical effects of the changing heart position) and before going to sleep (when the mind may be active but the brain has no visual input to work on).

The majority of symptomatic patients experience normal occasional ectopics that are generally benign. However, the development of ectopic activity may indicate an adverse prognosis (e.g. VT or AF after myocardial infarction [MI]). Knowledge of whether the patient has structural heart disease is crucial in risk stratification. If it is clear that the patient has significant structural heart disease, the presence of ventricular ectopics may require further cardiologic investigation.

Atrial fibrillation. In patients with AF, the ventricular rate may vary considerably and be very fast or very slow. The presence of AF in a patient complaining of dizziness or syncope should raise the possibility of intermittent severe bradycardias and needs further investigation.

Slow heart rate. A slow regular heart rate at around 40 bpm should alert you to the possibility of complete heart block. In sinus rhythm, irregular cannon waves (large A waves that occur when the right atrium contracts against a closed tricuspid valve) in the jugular venous pulse should help to confirm the diagnosis. Be aware, however, that sinus rhythm with bigeminal ventricular ectopy will give a slow regular pulse at the wrist.

Breathlessness and fatigue

Although many patients seem to notice every abnormal heart beat, other patients never notice any change in their heart rhythm. Persistent tachycardias may also produce symptoms because of hemodynamic consequence.

Over time, tachycardia itself may produce global left ventricular (LV) systolic impairment, a situation known as tachycardiomyopathy. Termination of the tachycardia and restoration of sinus rhythm leads to progressive improvement in LV performance. Although most commonly seen with atrial tachycardia, this phenomenon may also occur with inadequately controlled AF where ventricular rate control is poor.

Falls and syncope

Cardiac syncope is usually characterized by sudden and complete loss of consciousness for less than 1–2 minutes. This transient loss of consciousness must be distinguished from a trip or a fall. The history is therefore crucial, although it may be difficult in some cases, as often loss of consciousness results in amnesia, particularly in the elderly, and hence syncope is denied.

Cerebral blood flow depends on maintenance of blood pressure, which in turn is directly related to both cardiac output and peripheral vascular resistance such that a drop in either may be associated with a fall or a dizzy spell. Features that may help to clarify if blackout has a cardiac cause are detailed in Table 3.2. There may be a short prodromal phase of sweating, dizziness or a sensation of fainting, often lasting less than 30 seconds.

Although many patients are briefly disorientated on regaining consciousness, recovery is rapid and complete within a short period (usually minutes). It is unusual to have a prolonged period of unconsciousness (more than 5 minutes) with a cardiac cause, although witness description is notoriously unreliable. Patients are usually lucid quickly after an episode. Tonic–clonic seizure is uncommon but can occur because of cerebral anoxia. Incontinence is rare. The desire to sleep afterwards is also uncommon. Syncope is much more common than epilepsy.

Recurrent presyncope (the sensation patients describe when they feel they are about to lose consciousness) is common and may culminate in syncope over time. Presyncope occurs commonly in situations where the native cardiac pacemaker is impaired but not for long enough to produce syncope (e.g. sick sinus syndrome or carotid sinus hypersensitivity). Self-injury is variable. In some cases, symptoms may occur over many years before a diagnosis is made. In many cases, specific precipitating factors are uncommon.

Presyncope needs to be differentiated from dizziness, which can include vertigo.

Syncope in patients with known structural heart disease, particularly impaired LV function, carries a significantly worse prognosis with an increased risk of sudden death. These patients require urgent cardiologic investigation.

Differential diagnoses for causes of falls and blackouts are shown in
Table 3.4. Patients with cardiac syncope often do not remember the loss of

TABLE 3.2

Features of patient history that indicate a cardiac cause of blackout

- Sudden-onset/unheralded loss of consciousness
- Presence of structural heart disease (e.g. previous myocardial infarction or cardiac surgery)
  - impaired or poor left ventricular function
  - aortic stenosis
  - hypertrophic cardiomyopathy
  - pulmonary stenosis
  - pulmonary hypertension
  - pulmonary embolism
  - cardiac tumor
  - obstructed prosthetic valve
  - cardiac tamponade
- An arrhythmia (particularly if palpitations precede the blackouts)
- Prodromal symptoms (e.g. patients sometimes complain of a curtain coming down in their vision or a 'graying' of their visual fields)*
- Any triggers such as emotion, swallowing, micturition, coughing (e.g. syncope with micturition may indicate an inappropriate vagal response; syncope with noxious stimuli usually signifies a vasovagal or neurocardiogenic origin)
- Absence of features to suggest a fit (e.g. convulsions, incontinence, tongue-biting, post-blackout drowsiness); remember to ask witnesses **– remember that anoxia due to low blood pressure may masquerade as a tonic–clonic seizure**
- Age (new syncope in the elderly is more likely to be due to sick sinus syndrome or, less likely, carotid sinus hypersensitivity)
- Medication (Table 3.3)

*Vasovagal episodes often have prodromal symptoms such as nausea, sweating, chest pain and palpitations.

consciousness and hence only consider that they have had a fall. However, instances of sudden unheralded blackout without prodromal symptoms

TABLE 3.3

Medications that may contribute to falls and syncope

Antihypertensives	Heart-rate-slowing agents
• Beta-blockers	• Beta-blockers (used intermittently or long term)
• Vasodilators, including calcium-channel blockers (severe postural hypotension) and nitrate preparations	• Verapamil/diltiazem
• Prasozin	• Digoxin
• Thiazides	
• ACE inhibitors	
• Angiotensin-receptor blockers	

ACE, angiotensin-converting enzyme.

and with brief loss of consciousness are almost certainly cardiac in origin. Further investigations will help to ascertain whether the blackout has a cardiac cause.

Dizziness

This is a subjective symptom. Dizziness may encompass a number of pathologies including loss of balance or difficulty with gait. It is not often reliably associated with cardiac pathology.

Chest discomfort

This is usually not a feature of bradyarrhythmias but can be associated with tachyarrhythmias, both ventricular and supraventricular. However, pain is not usually an accepted feature of an arrhythmia. If the patient complains of pain then other conditions should be considered such as associated angina. It is common for anxious patients to complain of a sharp, left inframammary stabbing pain, but this is often innocuous.

Physical signs

Murmurs. Systolic murmurs may reflect aortic stenosis, a well-recognized cause of syncope, or hypertrophic cardiomyopathy (HCM). Diastolic murmurs are rare. Very rarely, intracardiac masses such as a myxoma (for

TABLE 3.4

Causes of falls and blackouts

Falls (i.e. no loss of consciousness)*

- Trips due to environmental issues (e.g. loose rugs, ice)
- Mechanical instability (e.g. arthritis, vertigo)

Transient loss of consciousness

- Cardiac syncope due to structural heart disease
  - aortic stenosis
  - hypertrophic cardiomyopathy
  - right ventricular cardiomyopathy
- Cardiac syncope due to arrhythmia
  - tachycardia (e.g. VT, polymorphic VT, Brugada syndrome, SVT)
  - bradycardia (e.g. AV block, sinus node disease)
- Cardiac syncope due to vascular causes
  - vasovagal syncope
  - carotid sinus hypersensitivity
  - situational (e.g. cough) syncope
  - postural orthostatic hypotension
  - postural orthostatic tachycardia syndrome (POTS)
- Epilepsy

Apparent loss of consciousness

- Psychogenic causes

*Need to be excluded in elderly patients who have a fall, because 30% of patients with syncope do not remember the loss of consciousness and hence only consider that they have had a fall.
AV, atrioventricular; SVT, supraventricular tachycardia; VT, ventricular tachycardia.

which the physical sign is a tumor plop on auscultation) or a thrombus may be present. Clinical heart failure may indicate significant LV dysfunction or valvular heart disease. A third or fourth heart sound may also reflect impaired LV function.

Sudden death

Arrhythmias can be fatal, at initial presentation or after persistent episodes. Some factors predict an increased risk of sudden death, including poor LV systolic function. It is generally accepted that an LV ejection fraction of less than 35% (normal is in excess of 50%) is associated with an increased risk of sudden arrhythmic death. Syncope in patients with known ischemic heart disease, previous MI or aortic valve disease carries a significantly adverse prognosis; these patients need urgent cardiologic investigation.

Other less common conditions that also predispose to sudden death include HCM (see page 122), Brugada syndrome (see page 120), Wolff–Parkinson–White (WPW) syndrome (see pages 16–20), the long-QT syndromes (see pages 117–20) and arrhythmogenic right ventricular dysplasia (see pages 121–2).

Who should be referred?

Symptomatic patients with:
- intrusive symptoms
- palpitations and ECG evidence of pre-excitation (WPW syndrome)
- syncope, or presyncope (see above)
- palpitations and known structural heart disease.

Patients with a combination of known structural heart disease and syncope or presyncope, with or without palpitations, should be referred urgently.

Asymptomatic patients. Arrhythmias are usually treated because symptoms interfere with a patient's quality of life. In certain situations it is crucial to know if treatment is warranted because of an adverse prognosis even if the patient is asymptomatic (Table 3.5).

TABLE 3.5

Indications for specialist referral in asymptomatic patients

- Ventricular pre-excitation (Wolff–Parkinson–White syndrome)
- Certain occupations (e.g. airline pilot, truck driver) with abnormal ECGs
- Atrial fibrillation
- Hypertrophic cardiomyopathy
- Family history of sudden cardiac death – long-QT syndrome, Brugada ECG (see pages 120–1), abnormal resting ECG

Key points – presenting signs and symptoms

- Patients with arrhythmias can present in a variety of ways.
- It is important to distinguish increased awareness of heart beat from true cardiac arrhythmias.
- Syncope with or without palpitations requires urgent referral.
- Patients with palpitations and known structural cardiac disease should also be referred urgently.

Key references

Benditt DG. Neurally mediated syncopal syndromes: pathophysiological concepts and clinical evaluation. *Pacing Clin Electrophysiol* 1997;20:572–84.

Petkar S, Cooper P, Fitzpatrick AP. How to avoid a misdiagnosis in patients presenting with transient loss of consciousness. *Postgrad Med J* 2006;82:630–41.

The problem of the intermittent fault

Like car mechanics faced with a car with an intermittent problem, physicians can adopt one of several approaches to finding the cause of intermittent palpitations:

- predicting it – by identifying features present between episodes that favor an arrhythmia as the cause
- waiting for it – and recording an attack when it happens
- provoking it – by bringing on the arrhythmia in a controlled way so that it can be studied.

The approach to take in patients with palpitations depends on the severity of the episode and the frequency of the attacks.

Predicting it

This is achieved by evaluation of the baseline abnormalities that may be present between episodes by history taking and examination.

History taking. Features of relevance include any history of previous infarction or cardiac surgery. In addition, any history to suggest the presence of structural heart disease, including hypertension or diabetes, makes an arrhythmia much more likely to be the cause of symptoms. A family history of sudden death is also relevant.

Clinical examination should be performed to look for evidence of structural heart disease, including murmur, heart failure and hypertension.

Electrocardiogram. A 12-lead ECG in an asymptomatic patient may reveal features such as pathological Q waves to indicate a previous myocardial infarction (MI) and thus structural disease, or may show more specific markers of arrhythmia risk such as ventricular pre-excitation, a long-QT interval or Brugada syndrome.

Referral for more detailed investigations to exclude structural heart disease may be necessary for some patients, particularly those with ventricular ectopics. Additional investigation may include an echocardiogram (cardiac ultrasound), which will give accurate information about the pumping action of the heart and the structure of the heart and valves.

Waiting for it – recording an episode

Recording of an ECG during symptoms is crucial to establishing the mechanism in a patient with palpitations. Modern digital devices offer much greater flexibility and better yield than early cassette-based recording devices but their use still requires careful planning. The clinical utility of 24-hour ambulatory ECG recording depends on several factors, but mainly on the frequency of episodes.

The frequency of symptoms will dictate the best investigation to carry out (Table 4.1). For example, a patient who presents with a sustained arrhythmia (perhaps at the first presentation) and is not hemodynamically compromised, requires a 12-lead ECG, which may have to be carried out at the local emergency unit. It is worth telling the patient that they should have an ECG done immediately on arrival, or provide them with an explanatory letter to present at the unit. The recording of an ECG during

TABLE 4.1

Frequency of episodes as an indication for choice of investigation

Frequency of episodes	Investigation
Very rare but sustained (hours)	• Observe pulse rate
	• Self-attendance at primary care clinic or hospital emergency department for a 12-lead ECG
Sustained	• 12-lead ECG during symptoms
Brief	
• Exercise related	• Exercise test
• Daily	• Holter (24-hour ambulatory recorder)
• Infrequent (less than once per week) but tolerated	• Patient-activated recorder
Infrequent (less than once per week) but severe (either intrusive symptoms or recurrent but infrequent syncope)	• Implantable loop recorder (see Figure 4.2)

symptoms saves a considerable amount of time and effort and will enable the correct diagnosis and management.

Types of recorders (continuous vs intermittent). The advantages and disadvantages of the three main types of recorder are summarized in Table 4.2.

Continuous Holter monitor. This can be attached via a strap worn over the shoulder or, more usually, it is carried on a belt; electrodes attached to the skin record the electrical activity of the heart (Figure 4.1). These monitors are often used for 24-hour recording but can be worn for up to 72 hours if required.

External loop recorder. The patient wears a device on the wrist or around the waist and presses a button on the device to record heart activity when symptoms are experienced.

Implantable loop recorder. The device (Figure 4.2) is inserted through a small incision (approximately 2 cm wide) in an area of the chest that yields the best signal from the heart, usually on the left mid-upper chest.

Provoking it – electrophysiological testing

Many patients, particularly those with severe or life-threatening arrhythmias, require provocative procedures. Treadmill exercise testing can be used to evaluate arrhythmias and is a useful option before electrophysiological (EP) testing, particularly in patients who describe arrhythmias under exercise conditions. Because the majority of human arrhythmias are re-entrant, EP testing has a high chance of unmasking a propensity for a regular arrhythmia. However, EP testing is not 100% sensitive, and often transient factors (e.g. emotions, changes in autonomic tone) that cannot be reproduced in the laboratory must be present for the arrhythmia to be provoked.

If a patient has had a documented cardiac arrhythmia, they usually have a continuing propensity for that arrhythmia. They have the potential (the substrate) for the arrhythmia but they do not have it all the time because they need a trigger to start it (usually random ectopic beats that allow re-entry to occur). By introducing electrical extra-stimuli into different chambers of the heart (equivalent to introducing ectopic beats but from a stimulator under controlled conditions), EP testing produces many possible triggers in a short time. During a diagnostic EP study,

TABLE 4.2

Types of recorder: advantages and disadvantages

Advantages	Disadvantages
Continuous Holter monitor	
• Not intrusive, so likely to be used • Long life • Cheap and widely available	• Requires long enough episode to allow recording • Low yield (2–4 of 100 cases are positive; a negative result does not exclude an arrhythmia) • Episode must be frequent (more than once daily) and well tolerated
Loop recorder	
• Activation of the device stops the ECG at that point and for a programmable period beforehand • Can be set to automatically record events (e.g. if heart rate exceeds a predetermined level)	• Electrodes may irritate the skin, or come off, reducing the quality of the recording • Electrodes need to be applied throughout continuous ECG recording, which may cause irritation
Implantable loop recorder	
• Long recording interval (36 months) • Ideal for very infrequent episodes • Automatic programmable recording period • New devices will be capable of being remotely interrogated using wireless technology	• Invasive • High yield in syncope • Expensive

pacing/recording electrodes are positioned within the heart, usually from the right femoral vein (Figure 4.3). Rarely, access via the jugular or subclavian veins is required. Wires are positioned at the high right atrial position (close to the sinus node), at the AV nodal area, within the coronary sinus and at the right ventricular apex. Small electrical impulses are then delivered through the wires at different sites (usually the atrium

43

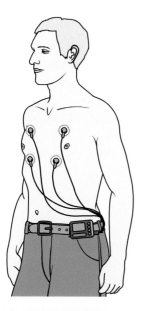

Figure 4.1 Continuous Holter monitor.

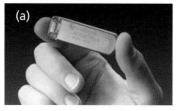

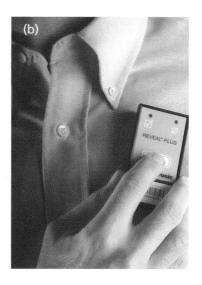

Figure 4.2 (a) Implantable loop recorder used for prolonged monitoring of cardiac rhythm; the recorder is inserted just below the skin over the heart, usually on the left mid-upper chest; (b) the patient can activate the recorder using a remote-control pad.

and ventricles) and the spread of these impulses through the heart defines any electrical abnormalities. The patient does not feel these impulses and is often awake during the procedure.

The impulses are carefully timed: first, a sequence of eight beats (known as the 'drive train' or S1) is delivered at a constant rate (typically

(a) 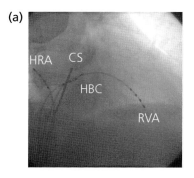 (b)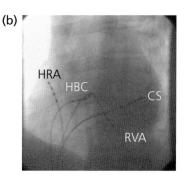

Figure 4.3 Radiographs of pacing/recording electrodes within the heart in (a) the right anterior oblique and (b) the left anterior oblique positions. (b) shows that the coronary sinus (CS) runs posteriorly, between the left atrium and ventricle. Each catheter has between 4 and 10 recording poles. HBC, His bundle catheter at the AV nodal area; HRA, high right atrium; RVA, right ventricular apex.

100 bpm) to stabilize the conduction properties of the heart. A ninth beat (S2) is then introduced earlier and earlier, to simulate an ectopic beat. The electrophysiologist analyzes what happens to the impulse as it spreads around the heart, until the impulse fails to conduct (the refractory period of the tissue) or an arrhythmia is produced. Once the electrical abnormality is defined, an ablation is performed to target the substrate.

For arrhythmias that do not have this re-entrant mechanism and cannot normally be initiated by the extra-stimulus technique (described above), a variety of other strategies to induce the arrhythmia can be tried, including administration of sympathetic nervous system stimulants such as isoprenaline (isoproterenol). Sometimes, however, the arrhythmia is completely non-inducible despite good documentation of the arrhythmia; catheter ablation generally cannot be performed in these cases.

The ability to record electrical activity within various chambers of the heart is a relatively new development, which, coupled with the therapeutic arm of catheter ablation, has transformed the management of cardiac arrhythmias.

What does electrophysiological testing involve? The procedure is usually performed under local anesthesia in a cardiac catheterization laboratory ('cath lab'); the patient may need to stay in hospital. EP testing has a high success rate (more than 90% in regular tachycardias) and a low complication rate.

Each EP study has three stages:
- preparation and instrumentation
- provocation of the arrhythmia and diagnosis
- catheter ablation (if appropriate).

Preparation and instrumentation. Patients should not eat or drink for up to 12 hours before the procedure. Antiarrhythmic medication must be stopped for 5 half-lives before the procedure; amiodarone has a prolonged half-life and therefore should be stopped 3 months before the procedure, or not at all. On the ward, staff will provide the patient with appropriate information, check consent and, if necessary, administer premedication. In the cath lab, an external defibrillator and the recording systems are connected to the patient. It usually takes about half an hour for the clinician to obtain vascular access and introduce the catheters.

Provocation of the arrhythmia. Patients may be fearful of catheter manipulation and should be reassured that moving catheters within the heart is not painful. However, the mechanical effect of having a wire in the heart can produce ectopics, which the patient may feel. Introducing electrical stimuli via the catheter is not painful and generally goes unnoticed. The arrhythmia may need to be initiated and terminated repeatedly.

Catheter ablation may be required once the diagnosis and location of the abnormality are clear. Catheter ablation is discussed in greater detail in Chapter 5 and the management sections of subsequent chapters.

What are the risks? The risks depend on the type of procedure being undertaken and the arrhythmia under study. Occasionally, the pre-procedural diagnosis is clear (e.g. with Wolff–Parkinson–White syndrome), but because ablation is now usually combined with a diagnostic EP study it is best to quote generic risk.

Who needs an electrophysiological study?

Although EP studies were previously considered essential to evaluate cardiac arrhythmias or syncope, they are now predominantly performed as part of a catheter ablation procedure for SVT or VT. EP studies are generally not indicated in patients with a LV ejection fraction (LVEF) of less than 30%, as these individuals are candidates for defibrillators, or in patients with syncope who have preserved LV function and a normal ECG, as these individuals are likely to receive a loop monitor. EP studies are usually performed in patients with syncope who have moderate LV dysfunction and a LVEF greater than 30%. They may also be indicated in selected patients with channelopathies.

Key points – investigation

- Performing an ECG (12-lead if possible) during symptoms is essential.
- The frequency of a patient's symptoms will determine the best non-invasive test to apply.
- Non-invasive monitoring can be performed repeatedly if needed.
- Electrophysiological (EP) testing was initially conceived to provoke and identify cardiac arrhythmias.
- Catheter ablation is generally now performed during the EP testing procedure.

Key references

DiMarco JP, Philbrick JT. Use of ambulatory electrocardiographic (Holter) monitoring. *Ann Intern Med* 1990;113:53–68.

Fogoros RN. *Electrophysiologic Testing*, 4th edn. WileyBlackwell, 2006.

Huang SK, Wiber DJ, eds. *Radiofrequency Catheter Ablation of Cardiac Arrhythmias: Basic Concepts and Clinical Applications*, 2nd edn. WileyBlackwell, 2002.

Jalife J, Delmar M, Anumonwo J et al., eds. *Basic Cardiac Electrophysiology for the Clinician*, 2nd edn. WileyBlackwell, 2009.

Josephson ME. *Clinical Cardiac Electrophysiology: Techniques and Interpretations*, 4th edn. Lippincott Williams & Wilkins, 2008.

Kinlay S, Leitch JW, Neil A et al. Cardiac event recorders yield more diagnoses and are more cost-effective than 48-hour Holter monitoring in patients with palpitations. A controlled clinical trial. *Ann Intern Med* 1996;124:16–20.

Krahn AD, Klein GJ, Yee R, Skanes AC. Randomized assessment of syncope trial: conventional diagnostic testing versus a prolonged monitoring strategy. *Circulation* 2001;104:46–51.

Optimal management of an arrhythmia is more likely if its mechanisms and natural history are fully understood (see Chapter 2). The patient's physical, psychological and biochemical status should be assessed thoroughly before considering treatment; thyroid function testing is mandatory.

Referral

It should be remembered that many arrhythmias – atrial and ventricular ectopy, supraventricular arrhythmias (SVTs), atrial flutter and atrial fibrillation (AF) – are not life-threatening, and patients should be reassured accordingly. However, many, if not most, patients will require the additional reassurance that referral to a cardiologist can provide. As a general rule, any patient with sustained/prolonged palpitations (of more than 30 seconds) should be referred.

General treatment principles

When making any decision about initiating treatment, care must be taken to assess the benefits and risks. Reasons for treatment may include:

- frequent and intrusive symptoms
- disabling symptoms (e.g. syncope, presyncope, chest pains, breathlessness), irrespective of frequency
- impaired quality of life
- significant comorbidity for which untreated arrhythmias may confer additional risk (e.g. development of AF in patients with hypertrophic cardiomyopathy [HCM], often leading to pulmonary edema or hemodynamic collapse)
- known structural heart disease
- high risk of sudden death.

The aim of treatment is to suppress symptoms, restore an acceptable quality of life and, if relevant, reduce the risk of sudden death. Intervention should provide long-term benefit and minimal risk. Before any intervention it is important to be sure that a genuine arrhythmia has been proven (see Chapter 4) and identified, and its short- and long-term significance evaluated. This will help to determine whether treatment is required, and what the safest and most effective treatment is. The options for treatment are:

- reassurance only (no active treatment)
- pharmacological treatment (antiarrhythmic drug therapy)
- non-pharmacological interventions (direct-current [DC] cardioversion, radiofrequency or cryoablation, pacemaker, surgery).

No intervention

Some arrhythmias do not require any intervention; for example, primary care physicians can manage most patients with symptomatic palpitations that are due to increased awareness of the heart beat only. When deciding to provide explanation and reassurance only, the physician must be certain that the patient's heart is structurally normal. This can be determined by a clinical examination and a normal 12-lead ECG (see Chapter 4). An echocardiogram may also be necessary for a few patients with resistant or longstanding symptoms. Table 5.1 lists the features to explain to patients with normal ectopic beats.

Atrial ectopy is a benign condition and it is rare for patients to be aware of just atrial ectopic beats. Provided there is no structural heart defect

TABLE 5.1

Reassurances to give to patients with normal ectopic beats

- Benign prognosis – not related to sudden death
- Very common
- Often the trigger is unknown but increased awareness may prolong symptoms
- Particularly often noticed at rest
- Suppressed by exercise
- Often occur in clusters (bigeminy)
- Documentation may be helpful though not always possible
- Brought on by emotional stress (and, conversely, ectopy can cause stress)

(normal resting ECG, clinical examination and normal thyroid function tests are usually sufficient evidence), nothing further is required. There is no convincing evidence that suppressing atrial ectopy prevents the onset of atrial arrhythmias or AF with time.

Ventricular ectopy. A small but important minority of patients are aware of ventricular ectopic beats. Symptoms are often variable and persistent despite reassurances. Periods of emotional stress are often associated with relapse and significant symptoms.

In the absence of a structural heart defect (a normal resting ECG and clinical examination may be sufficient, although an echocardiogram is advised), such ectopics are generally benign. They do not shorten life span and strong reassurance is the main form of management. Occasionally, cognitive therapy is required. Long-term antiarrhythmic therapy can usually be avoided. In many patients, however, quality of life can be severely adversely affected. If treatment is deemed necessary and the patient cannot be simply reassured, then beta-blockers may be beneficial. They are safe in the long term and rarely produce dangerous or proarrhythmic side effects.

In the presence of a structural heart defect, ventricular ectopics have a more sinister outlook. These patients need further investigation – particularly if left ventricular (LV) function is impaired. Such patients may have an increased risk of sudden death and require referral to a cardiologist. An echocardiogram is required in the assessment of these patients.

Sinus tachycardias rarely require treatment. There is nearly always an underlying cause that must be looked for, such as anemia, thyrotoxicosis, sepsis, pregnancy, anxiety or hypovolemia.

Pharmacological treatment
Classification of drugs. Historically, antiarrhythmic drugs have been classified by their action at cellular level; although useful as a starting point, this requires extrapolation to specific arrhythmias. The Vaughan-Williams classification is the most frequently used system of determining drug effect and action. Drugs often fit into more than one group, which can make their practical application confusing. A simplified version of this classification is shown in Table 5.2.

TABLE 5.2

Vaughan-Williams classification of antiarrhythmic drugs

Mechanism of action	Main site of action	Examples
Class 1		
Fast sodium-channel blocker, increases APD	Atria, Ventricles Accessory pathways	Class 1a: Quinidine*, Procainamide[†], Disopyramide, Ajmaline[‡]
		Class 1b: Lidocaine, Mexiletine*
		Class 1c: Flecainide, Propafenone
Class 2		
Blocks sympathetic beta-receptors	Sinus and AV nodes	Beta-blockers
Class 3		
Blocks potassium channels, increases APD	Atria, AV node, His-Purkinje fibers, Ventricles, Accessory pathways	Amiodarone, Sotalol, Ibutilide i.v.[†], Dofetilide*, Dronedarone
Class 4		
Blocks slow calcium channels	AV node	Adenosine (i.v. only), Verapamil, Diltiazem

*Not available in the UK.
[†]USA only.
[‡]Not available in the USA.
APD, action potential duration – a longer APD generally slows cardiac conduction; AV, atrioventricular; i.v. intravenous.

Generic side effects. All antiarrhythmic drugs have side effects, most of which are drug specific. However, antiarrhythmic drugs have two generic side effects – proarrhythmia and negative inotropism.

Proarrhythmia. Every antiarrhythmic drug has the potential to worsen the arrhythmia being treated by increasing either the frequency or the severity of the arrhythmia, or by producing a different arrhythmia (which could be fatal). The risk of proarrhythmia increases in the presence of impaired LV function (Figure 5.1). Class 1 drugs such as flecainide and propafenone should only be used where LV function is normal. Proarrhythmia may be potentiated at fast or slow heart rates or during myocardial ischemia, and in the presence of hypo- or hyperkalemia.

Negative inotropism. By slowing parts, or all, of the conducting pathways, antiarrhythmic drugs have the potential to suppress myocardial contractility. Where LV function is normal this rarely has any sequelae or clinical effects. Where myocardial function is depressed, however, antiarrhythmic therapy can have serious deleterious effects such as worsening heart failure, proarrhythmia and increased mortality risk. Many scientific reports have shown arrhythmia suppression but at the expense of increased mortality.

The extent to which drugs are negatively inotropic varies (Figure 5.2). Class 1 drugs (flecainide/propafenone) and the beta-blocker sotalol should be avoided where LV function is impaired (ejection fraction < 35%). If in doubt, cardiologic assessment is mandatory.

Maintenance of sinus rhythm. The aim of antiarrhythmic drug therapy is to suppress the frequency of paroxysmal arrhythmias. The drugs are not curative, so treatment tends to be life long and the drugs must be taken daily (some of them three times daily). No drug taken orally is effective immediately, although some drugs can be useful when taken as soon as the arrhythmia begins. In cases where attacks are very infrequent, a small dose of a drug may be taken at the onset of symptoms (the so-called 'pill in the pocket' approach). However, this should not be repeated continuously if the arrhythmia fails to terminate, as pretreatment with a drug may complicate any subsequent aggressive treatment such as DC conversion in hospital. Table 5.3 summarizes the drugs that can be used for specific arrhythmias.

In pregnancy and breastfeeding, these agents need to be individualized. Ablation is the treatment of choice in young women, as drug use may be too risky if they wish to conceive.

Cardioversion. The development of new drugs has increased the popularity of pharmacological cardioversion, although some disadvantages persist, including the risk of drug-induced *torsades de*

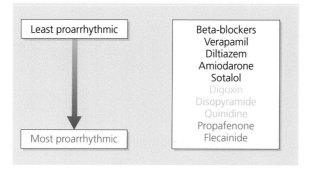

Figure 5.1 Relative proarrhythmic effects of antiarrhythmic drugs.

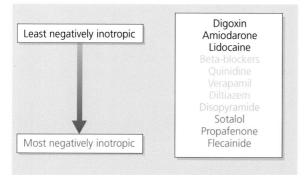

Figure 5.2 Relative inotropic effects of antiarrhythmic drugs.

pointes and other serious ventricular arrhythmias. Pharmacological cardioversion is less effective than electrical cardioversion but does not require conscious sedation or anesthesia.

A frequent issue is whether antiarrhythmic drug therapy should be started in hospital or on an outpatient basis. With the exception of low-dose oral amiodarone, virtually all studies of pharmacological cardioversion have been limited to hospitalized patients.

Non-pharmacological interventions

Direct-current cardioversion involves the external application of an electric shock that is synchronized with the intrinsic QRS activity of the heart so that it does not coincide with the vulnerable phase of the cardiac cycle (the T wave). As a result, it is a safe and effective treatment for many arrhythmias. DC cardioversion can be used in an emergency or electively.

The procedure. Elective DC cardioversion is performed with the patient having fasted and under conscious sedation or, preferably, full anesthesia.

53

TABLE 5.3

Drug options for different types of arrhythmia

Sinus tachycardia	SVT (AVRT) using a concealed AP	SVT (AVRT) with overt pre-excitation (e.g. WPW syndrome)	AVNRT / Junctional tachycardia	Atrial fibrillation; Atrial flutter; Atrial tachycardia	Ventricular tachycardia
Possible underlying cause: anemia, fever, sepsis, shock, hypovolemia or thyrotoxicosis Often requires no treatment	*At AV node:* Beta-blockade, calcium-channel blockers *At AP:* Flecainide Propafenone Sotalol Amiodarone Disopyramide	*At AP:* Flecainide Propafenone Sotalol Amiodarone *At AV node:* Avoid all AV-blocking drugs	Vagal maneuvers Adenosine (i.v.) Verapamil Diltiazem Flecainide Beta-blockers Digoxin	*Cardioversion to SR:* Amiodarone Disopyramide Flecainide *At AV node:* Verapamil Diltiazem Digoxin Beta-blockade *Prevention:* Amiodarone Flecainide Propafenone Disopyramide Quinidine	*Termination:* Lidocaine (lignocaine) Amiodarone *Prevention:* Amiodarone Beta-blockers ± in combination Sotalol

AP, accessory pathway; AV, atrioventricular; AVNRT, atrioventricular nodal re-entrant tachycardia; AVRT, atrioventricular re-entrant tachycardia; SR, sinus rhythm; SVT, supraventricular tachycardia; WPW, Wolff–Parkinson–White.

The use of short-acting anesthesia allows cardioversion to be performed in a day-case setting, as patients usually recover rapidly after the procedure.

Electrical cardioversion is safe in patients with implanted pacemakers or defibrillators provided appropriate precautions are taken. The shock should be given as far from the device as possible and not directly over the generator, using the lowest effective energy.

Relapses. Sinus rhythm can be restored in a substantial proportion of, if not all, patients by DC cardioversion, but the rate of relapse will depend on the underlying arrhythmia.

Risks. Electrical cardioversion can precipitate VF if the shock is not synchronized to the R wave. Pharmacological intervention can be associated with bradycardias, serious pauses or ventricular arrhythmias following conversion to sinus rhythm.

Thromboembolic events have been reported in 1–7% of patients with AF who do not receive anticoagulation before cardioversion, but the risk is very low in adequately anticoagulated patients. Anticoagulation needs to be maintained for at least 3–4 weeks after cardioversion, because a return to full atrial contraction may be delayed and the risk of thromboembolism remains. The risk of thromboembolism or stroke is similar with pharmacological and electrical cardioversion, and anticoagulation is the same for both methods (see Chapter 8).

Various brief arrhythmias may arise, especially ventricular and supraventricular premature beats, bradycardia and short periods of sinus arrest. Sinus arrest occurs more frequently in patients who have received multiple antiarrhythmic agents at the time of cardioversion. VT and VF can be precipitated in patients with hypokalemia or digitalis intoxication. Ideally, digoxin should be stopped for 48 hours before cardioversion. Transient ST-segment elevation can appear on the ECG after cardioversion and blood levels of creatine kinase-MB can rise without significant demonstrable myocardial damage.

Radiofrequency ablation (RFA, or catheter ablation) of accessory pathways has revolutionized the management of arrhythmias, many of which are curable using this technique. RFA has also established new concepts and greater understanding of the anatomic substrates and mechanisms of arrhythmias. It has proved so successful in the treatment of accessory pathways that its benefit has been extended to other arrhythmias

55

including atrioventricular nodal re-entrant tachycardia (AVNRT; junctional tachycardias), atrial flutter, ventricular arrhythmias and, more recently, AF. Open heart surgery for the ablation of accessory pathways is rarely performed nowadays. Indications for RFA are listed in Table 5.4.

The procedure. RFA is usually performed at a single sitting after the diagnostic electrophysiological (EP) study (see pages 46–7). General anesthesia is rarely required. RFA uses energy similar to that used in surgical diathermy. Local heating up to 70°C causes irreversible tissue damage, localized to within 3–5 mm of the catheter tip; accurate mapping is therefore critical. Catheters are steerable with a modified tip that can safely reach every chamber of the heart (Figure 5.3).

Success rates are high (see below), recurrence is uncommon, the arrhythmia is often cured and lifelong drug therapy is no longer required.

Patients should not be aware of any sustained palpitations after RFA, but may become aware of ectopic beats. As they have had palpitations for many years they are attuned to the nature of their heart beat. With the substrate removed during ablation, patients are left with the trigger only, and feel as if the arrhythmia is about to start even though it cannot. These symptoms often last for some time after the ablation, occasionally for years. Patients can be reassured that treatment is rarely required.

TABLE 5.4

Usual indications for radiofrequency (catheter) ablation

- Symptomatic patient
- Failure or intolerance of medication
- Patient unwilling to take, or unable to afford, long-term medical therapy, or preference for non-pharmacological approach
- Woman of child-bearing age who does not use contraception or who wishes to start a family
- Ventricular ectopics with the characteristic morphology of origin from the right ventricular outflow tract (see Figure 9.2)
- VT in patients with CAD who have received shocks from their ICD in spite of antiarrhythmic therapy

CAD, coronary artery disease; ICD, implantable cardioverter defibrillator.

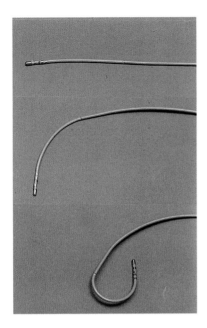

Figure 5.3 A radiofrequency ablation catheter showing the modified deflectable tip, which allows the catheter to be positioned virtually anywhere in the heart.

Complications are shown in Table 5.5. There is also a risk of radiation exposure, predominantly associated with complex ablation procedures (AF, VT). The degree of exposure relates to the patient's weight and the type of fluoroscopic and mapping systems used (see pages 99–100).

Ablation of accessory pathways. RFA can be used for both overt pre-excitation and concealed pathways (see pages 16–20). For accessory pathways as a whole, RFA is successful in 95% of cases as a first procedure. The procedure can always be repeated and is then usually completely successful.

The aim is to ablate the insertion site, usually within the atrium. Ablating this site, rather than the ventricular insertion, is thought to be safer and easier because of the thinness of the atrial wall. The left atrium can be approached in two ways: the transaortic retrograde approach via the femoral artery and the transseptal puncture approach (see Figure 8.8), through the intra-atrial septum.

Indications for RFA of accessory pathways are:
- patients in whom medical treatment has failed (although many cardiologists are now advocating RFA as first-line treatment given the safety profile of the procedure)

TABLE 5.5

Complications of radiofrequency ablation

Major	
Overall / none	3% / 97%
Permanent pacemaker*	1%
Myocardial infarction	0.1%
Thromboembolic stroke	0.2%
Tamponade	0.5%
Death	0.3%

Minor	
Overall	8%
Vascular – hematoma	3%
Transient atrioventricular block	2%
Pericardial effusion	2%
Pericarditis	0.4%

*Especially after ablation of atrioventricular nodal re-entrant tachycardia.
Adapted from data in Cappato R. *J Am Coll Cardiol* 2009;53:1798–803;
Hindricks G. *Eur Heart J* 1993;14:1644–53; Spragg D. *J Cardiovasc Electrophysiol*
2008;19:627–31.

- women of child-bearing age
- patients who have been resuscitated from sudden death (from a documented episode of VF) and where a delta wave is present on the surface ECG (see Figure 2.2).

Ablation of concealed pathways. These are mapped in the same manner as accessory pathways except that the pathway position is only manifest during constant ventricular pacing or during SVT, so the RF energy has to be delivered while pacing or during tachycardia. In these cases the time taken for the pacing impulse to go from the ventricle to the atrium (the VA time) is measured; the pathway position corresponds to the point at which the VA time is shortest. The VA time suddenly lengthens during successful ablation, indicating that the aberrant pathway has been destroyed (Figure 5.4). If RFA is performed during SVT, typically, the tachycardia stops suddenly and the patient returns to sinus rhythm.

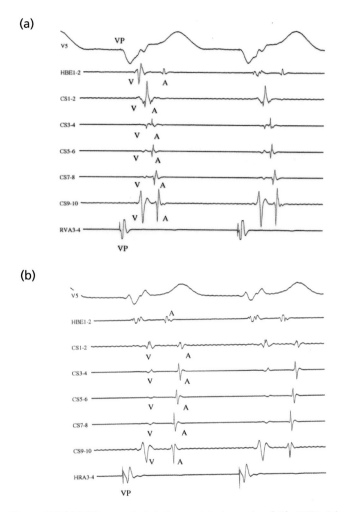

Figure 5.4 (a) ECGs recorded during ventricular pacing (VP). HBE1–2 is the bipolar ECG recorded from the His Bundle. CS1–2, 3–4, 5–6, 7–8 and 9–10 are bipolar ECGs recorded from a multielectrode catheter within the coronary sinus (CS) vein. CS1–2 represents the distal CS recording from the left side of the heart, while CS9–10 represents the proximal recording near the AV node. During ventricular pacing, the time between the atrial and ventricular signals (the VA time) is very short, being shortest in CS1–2, thereby revealing the position of the pathway. (b) Following ablation, the VA time becomes much longer, confirming that the pathway has been destroyed and depolarization of the atria from the ventricles is now passing retrogradely through the AV node.

Ablation for AVNRT (junctional tachycardia). Ablation of the slow pathway has a better safety profile and is now the procedure of choice. A feared complication is irreversible complete heart block but this is rare (1% at most). Nevertheless, as many of these patients are young, the risk of heart block and the need for a permanent pacemaker must be discussed in detail beforehand.

Cryoablation. While RFA produces cell fulguration or a localized burn, cryoablation freezes the tissues at the catheter tip. Tissues can be 'pre-frozen' before cell death occurs, and if necessary cryoablation can be interrupted during this period of pre-freezing to allow warming of the tissues and reversal of the effects of ablation. Thus, in select circumstances such as ablation near the AV node, for certain types of accessory pathway or during AVNRT, cryoablation may be a safer procedure than RFA. However, cryoablation is associated with a higher relapse rate than RFA, as pathway conduction may recover after the procedure. In general, RFA produces better long-term outcomes.

Endocardial versus epicardial ablation. In most cases the arrhythmic substrate lies within reach of the endocardial surface. However, occasionally the substrate lies in the epicardial tissues. This is increasingly being recognized, particularly for ventricular arrhythmias, although, rarely, accessory pathways can lie on the outer surface of the heart. These arrhythmias can be treated by placing the ablation/mapping catheters within the epicardial space, which is accessed percutaneously via the subxiphoid approach. Although this can be a highly successful treatment for epicardial arrhythmias, it involves small but significant risks.

Risk stratification in Wolff–Parkinson–White syndrome

Patients with pre-excitation have a very small risk of sudden death, which must be considered even in asymptomatic individuals. The risk is related to the development of AF, which can occur spontaneously or following the onset of an SVT. If rapid impulses in the atria pass exclusively over the accessory pathway without slowing, a rapid ventricular rate may develop, resulting in VF.

Features that favor low-risk WPW syndrome are:
- intermittent pre-excitation
- pre-excitation that disappears with exercise, or with intravenous ajmaline (in Europe) or intravenous procainamide (in the USA), class 1 antiarrhythmic drugs with potent sodium-channel blocking effects.

Lifestyle considerations

Taking all the options discussed above into account, the final management plan will depend on the individual's circumstances and consideration of the patient's lifestyle.

Age per se is not a contraindication to catheter ablation – results are similar in patients in their eighties to those in their teens. Sadly, many elderly patients attribute their apparent slowing up or limitation to their age rather than any arrhythmia.

Specific triggers, such as alcohol or caffeine, can sometimes be identified and avoidance of these can effectively suppress episodes of arrhythmia in some patients, although this is infrequent. For most patients, exercise is to be encouraged but in some (e.g. those with right ventricular outflow tract [RVOT] tachycardia or HCM) strenuous exercise is contraindicated. Elite endurance athletes usually undergo major changes to the structure and autonomic regulation of their hearts and may develop automatic arrhythmias (e.g. AF or RVOT) or produce changes that resemble right ventricular dysplasia. Detraining (if it is acceptable to the patient) will often correct the arrhythmia.

Ultimately, the decision to undertake catheter ablation will be based not only on the severity of the arrhythmia, but also the fear and uncertainty of an episode and the side effects of any medication (e.g. sun intolerance to amiodarone) and the restriction this may pose on the patient's lifestyle.

Key points – management principles

- Radiofrequency (catheter) ablation can cure many types of arrhythmia.
- Drug therapy can be useful to suppress symptoms initially but is not curative.
- Symptomatic patients should be considered for ablative therapy.

Definition

Supraventricular tachycardia (SVT) is a general term describing any rapid heart rate that originates above the ventricles. Although this can include atrial fibrillation (AF) and atrial flutter, as electrophysiology has improved our knowledge of mechanisms, it is now generally accepted that SVTs mean re-entrant arrhythmias where the main driver lies in the atria: approximately 60% are atrioventricular nodal re-entrant tachycardia (AVNRT; also known as junctional tachycardia), 30% are atrioventricular re-entrant tachycardia (AVRT) and 10% are atrial tachycardia.

Atrial tachycardia may be micro re-entrant (initiated and terminated by extrastimuli) or more commonly automatic (and localized) and typically influenced by autonomic tone. Atrial tachycardias may arise from anywhere in the atria but the most common sites are in the right atrium along the crista terminalis (including the base of the atrial appendage) and in the left atrium in the pulmonary veins and around the mitral valve.

SVTs are not usually life-threatening, although they can be in rare circumstances.

Epidemiology

SVTs usually occur in young, otherwise healthy, adults but can be seen at any age. There are surprisingly few data on the incidence of SVTs in the general population. In the USA the prevalence is estimated to be 2.25 per 1000 persons, with an incidence of 35 per 100 000 person-years. This equates to approximately 89 000 new cases per year and a total of about 570 000 people with SVTs in the USA at any time; the rate of presentation to the emergency room with a definite SVT was 0.05% per year over an 11-year period. Thus, SVTs are relatively infrequent.

Diagnosis

ECG. The characteristic feature is usually a regular narrow QRS complex on the surface ECG during symptoms (Figure 6.1). Wide-complex SVTs do occur but are considerably less common. The P wave morphology can help to localize the atrial origin of the tachycardia. This feature may not be

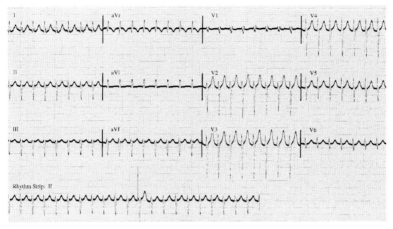

Figure 6.1 ECG trace of a narrow QRS complex, indicating a SVT.

initially evident but the nature of the arrhythmia can often be unmasked by producing temporary AV block by either vagal stimulation (e.g. carotid sinus massage) or administration of adenosine (see page 111). Some atrial tachycardias are adenosine sensitive and may terminate rather than reveal that the AV node is not required for the arrhythmia. Termination of a narrow-QRS tachycardia after intravenous administration of adenosine is often diagnostic of a tachycardia that involves the AV node (e.g. AVNRT) or a tachycardia mediated by an accessory pathway, but it does not exclude an atrial tachycardia.

Clinical presentation. Characteristically, patients complain of sudden onset of rapid palpitations. Often these feel regular but this is not always a reliable description, as patients often have difficulty telling the difference between a regular and irregular rhythm, particularly when the heart rate is fast. Associated symptoms are:

- sudden onset – sometimes the patient is aware of a brief run of ectopy before the tachycardia starts
- sudden offset
- chest pain (sometimes anginal like)
- shortness of breath
- faintness or presyncope (faintness may occur immediately at the onset or after the arrhythmia has been running for a while)
- sweating and nausea.

63

Syncope is uncommon. Very rarely, but often in younger patients, a persistent atrial tachycardia may present as heart failure.

Management

No intervention. If symptoms are infrequent and non-intrusive (e.g. once or twice a year), and provided the diagnosis is confirmed, no treatment may be indicated and the patient can be reassured. The patient can be given the options available, so that any increase in symptom frequency can be dealt with immediately. This advice applies only in the absence of ventricular pre-excitation (as in Wolff–Parkinson–White [WPW] syndrome). Patients who also have ventricular pre-excitation should be referred to a cardiologist for assessment of risk.

Vagal maneuvers. The arrhythmia can be terminated by vagal maneuvers, which effect selective slowing of conduction through the AV node (Table 6.1). These maneuvers work variably – not at all in some patients – but should be tried as they are low risk and simple to perform.

The safest and easiest to teach is the Valsalva maneuver, whereby the patient strains against a closed glottis. This can be achieved by asking the patient to imagine they are straining at stool or blowing hard with the mouth closed while pinching the nose. The forced expiration is maintained for 10 seconds and the tachycardia may terminate in the vagal phase on release of the breath hold.

TABLE 6.1

Vagal maneuvers

- Valsalva maneuver (see text)
- Straining
- Carotid sinus massage – one side at a time while the patient is supine
- Ice-cold drink/cold spoon down the back
- Changes in posture – standing up quickly or bending over

Note: Eyeball massage is contraindicated and dangerous and can result in eye damage.

Pharmacological treatment. As discussed above, these arrhythmias use an accessory pathway (AVRT), or in the case of AVNRT a slow pathway, as part of the tachycardia in addition to the AV node (see Chapter 2). The tachycardia can be terminated by slowing conduction through the AV node and/or the pathway. Usually, antegrade depolarization of the ventricle occurs over the AV node. The QRS complexes are therefore narrow during tachycardia. However, if the patient has an underlying bundle branch block, or if the tachycardia is associated with development of bundle branch block, the QRS may be wide.

Flecainide acetate is effective for the termination of arrhythmias and for suppressing recurrence. It has a particular action on the accessory pathway, slowing conduction and reducing its ability to sustain an arrhythmia. Flecainide should be avoided in patients with impaired left ventricular (LV) function or clinical heart failure, as the risk of proarrhythmia increases significantly in the presence of an impaired left ventricle. In these circumstances, an SVT can be converted to a potentially fatal arrhythmia – ventricular tachycardia (VT, which can be incessant) or recurrent ventricular fibrillation (VF). These risks are minimal when LV function is normal, as in the majority of patients with SVTs. The usual oral dose of flecainide is 100 mg twice daily, although occasionally 50 mg twice daily is effective. The dose can be increased under exceptional circumstances to 100 mg three times daily or 150 mg twice daily, but only with cardiologic advice.

Beta-blockers can be helpful but are less effective at suppressing arrhythmia recurrence. However, a combination of flecainide and a small dose of a beta-blocker can be effective.

Propafenone has partial beta-blocking actions and is not recommended in patients with at least moderate asthma. It requires the same precautions as flecainide, as they are both in the same Vaughan-Williams class (see Table 5.2). Propafenone should be avoided in any patient with impaired LV function. The usual dosage is 150 mg three times daily.

Sotalol also has partial beta-blocking actions and should be avoided in patients with any degree of asthma. Treatment should be started at 40–80 mg twice daily and increased gradually. The maximum dosage is 320 mg twice daily; however, if 160 mg is ineffective, therapy should be changed as it is unlikely that a greater dose will be effective. Sotalol should be used with great caution in the presence of heart failure and is generally

65

avoided in the elderly because of renal excretion. It is also used with caution in women in view of the risks of *torsades de pointes*.

Amiodarone. With the advent of non-pharmacological therapies, amiodarone for SVT should only be used as a last resort and with cardiologic guidance.

Adenosine. Intravenous administration of adenosine as a rapid bolus via a large vein is standard treatment for regular narrow-QRS tachycardias and has a high degree of success. Patients should be warned that they will experience a flush and possibly chest pain following the injection. The effect is usually quite dramatic but disappears within a few seconds. Occasionally, treatment with adenosine may reinitiate the arrhythmia, in which case longer-term suppressive therapy must be considered. AF may also be provoked.

Drugs to be avoided

In the normal heart. Any drug that exerts its major action by blocking the AV node should be avoided in pre-excitation syndromes, as in the WPW syndrome; such agents include verapamil, diltiazem and digoxin. None of these drugs alters accessory pathway function, so by blocking the AV node all conduction to the ventricles is likely to occur over the pathway. As SVTs can sometimes degenerate to AF (see Chapter 8) this can cause transmission of a rapid atrial rate to the ventricles, leading to VF. Many drugs that affect accessory pathway conduction also affect the AV node but it is the differential effect that is important.

In the damaged heart. Only beta-blockers and amiodarone have an acceptable safety profile in patients with LV damage; flecainide, propafenone and sotalol must be avoided. Serious consideration should be given to non-pharmacological therapies, sooner rather than later.

Non-pharmacological interventions

Direct-current (DC) cardioversion for an SVT is uncommon and is only used where intravenous therapy has been ineffective.

Occasionally, patients may have such a fast tachycardia that blood pressure is compromised and urgent DC cardioversion may be appropriate. Anesthesia or sedation is necessary unless the patient is unconscious.

Radiofrequency (catheter) ablation (RFA), as described in Chapter 5, is successful in 95% of cases as a first procedure for AVNRT or AVRT. In atrial tachycardia the success rates are lower (60–80%), depending on the inducibility and mapping. If necessary, the procedure can be repeated and is then usually completely successful. Indications for RFA are listed in Table 5.4. It is rare that RFA needs to be applied acutely.

Prognosis

The prognosis for patients with SVTs is excellent. Rarely, if an atrial tachycardia becomes incessant it may cause cardiac failure due to a tachycardiomyopathy.

Key points – supraventricular arrhythmias

- Where ventricular pre-excitation is found incidentally on ECG (e.g. patients with Wolff–Parkinson–White [WPW] syndrome), referral for cardiologic assessment and risk profiling is recommended. Regular antiarrhythmic therapy is not advised in asymptomatic cases.
- In symptomatic patients with WPW syndrome, even if symptoms are minimal, antiarrhythmia medication is advised and an assessment for ablation should be made.
- First-line treatment in the presence of normal ventricular function is catheter ablation or antiarrhythmic drug use (flecainide, propafenone or sotalol).

Key references

Murman DH, McDonald AJ, Pelletier AJ, Camargo CA Jr. U.S. emergency department visits for supraventricular tachycardia, 1993–2003. *Acad Emerg Med* 2007;14:578–81.

Orejarena LA, Vidaillet H Jr, DeStefano F et al. Paroxysmal supraventricular tachycardia in the general population. *J Am Coll Cardiol* 1998;31:150–7.

7 Atrial flutter

Definition
Typical atrial flutter is a macro-entrant atrial rhythm, rotating counterclockwise, occasionally clockwise, within the right atrium (see Figure 2.7). Most common is a circuit confined to the anterior portion of the right atrium with a 2:1 atrioventricular (AV) block – an atrial rate of 300 bpm and a regular ventricular response of 150 bpm related directly to the atrial rate. A QRS rate of exactly 150 bpm should raise suspicion of atrial flutter.

Epidemiology
Other than atrial fibrillation (AF), atrial flutter is the most common arrhythmia seen by cardiologists. Patients who have had AF may present with atypical atrial flutter at a later stage; patients who have had congenital abnormalities corrected at an early age may present with atypical atrial flutter up to 10–20 years later.

Causes
In typical atrial flutter, the circuit is critically dependent on an area of slow conduction known as the cavotricuspid isthmus (see Figure 2.7). Other rarer atypical forms occur, particularly in patients with scarring in the atrium (e.g. after radiofrequency ablation [RFA] or previous heart surgery).

Diagnosis
ECG. Atrial flutter typically has a saw-tooth appearance of flutter waves on the baseline in the 12-lead ECG (see Figure 2.7).

Clinical presentation. Atrial flutter can be aysmptomatic or may present with breathlessness, tiredness or frank heart failure. Persistent palpitations may be a feature.

Management
Anticoagulation therapy is based on the same risk factors as those for AF (see Chapter 8, pages 81–3 and 104–7).

Pharmacological treatment. In acute cases, cardioversion can be performed with intravenous ibutilide, or, if there is no structural heart disease, a class 1c antiarrhythmic agent, such as flecainide or propafenone, combined with a beta-blocker. Intravenous flecainide alone is sometimes used in Europe (but not in the USA) to slow conduction in the flutter circuit more than in the AV node itself. However, in some cases this may slow the atrial rate from 300 to 200 bpm and may allow the AV node to conduct in a 1:1 fashion, producing a paradoxical increase in the ventricular rate to 200 bpm, which may be associated with hemodynamic compromise; flecainide is often combined with a beta-blocker to prevent the flutter being conducted to the ventricle in this 1:1 manner. The same principle applies for both intravenous and oral flecainide.

Oral sotalol is often used in patients with atrial flutter, as it has the combined action of an antiarrhythmic and a beta-blocker, but QT considerations and renal excretion limit its use in women and the elderly. In the chronic setting, atrial flutter often responds poorly to drug therapy. AV nodal-blocking drugs slow the ventricular response.

Direct-current (DC) cardioversion is highly effective for atrial flutter. However, persistent atrial flutter (lasting longer than 48 hours) is associated with significant embolic risk, and management before cardioversion should be as for patients with AF – treatment with oral anticoagulant therapy (warfarin) for 4 weeks before cardioversion and for at least 1 month afterwards (see Chapter 8). Alternatively, a transesophageal echocardiogram can be performed in patients who are not taking warfarin, or in whom serial measurements of the international normalized ratio (INR) over a month have not been documented, to exclude left atrial thrombus and enable immediate cardioversion. Patients are then started, or continued, on warfarin, while heparin or low-molecular-weight heparin is given until the INR is greater than 2, continuing warfarin for 1 month or more.

In the acute setting, flutter often converts with a low-energy shock of about 50 J, sometimes as low as 25 J.

Radiofrequency (catheter) ablation is recommended for long-term treatment. RFA restores sinus rhythm by creating a linear destructive lesion, across which the circulating depolarizing wavefront cannot pass.

69

This is known as a line of block and is usually created at the inferior wall of the right atrium (Figure 7.1). This technique is in contrast to the ablation of accessory or slow pathways, which require highly localized lesions. The procedure can be performed during constant atrial flutter or in sinus rhythm with pacing from the atrium or coronary sinus. Success rates are greater than 90% in most centers.

The cavotricuspid isthmus is not smooth throughout its length and has regions of thick muscle bundles. Ablation of these areas is best achieved with technology capable of producing deep lesions, such as large-tip or cooled radiofrequency energy. Newer techniques involving computerized mapping of the atria and catheter position are improving overall success.

Indications. Most centers are now performing ablation as first-line treatment.

Complications. Apart from the usual complications associated with instrumentation of the venous circulation, heart block or cardiac tamponade are rarely reported.

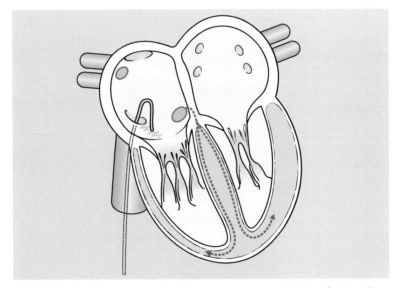

Figure 7.1 Ablation of atrial flutter. The catheter is placed in the inferior wall of the right atrium and slowly dragged back to the junction of the inferior vena cava with the atrial wall. Signals are recorded continuously from the catheter tip during the procedure.

Prognosis

After ablation, the prognosis for patients with typical atrial flutter is excellent. In patients with atypical atrial flutter recurrences are more common because of scarring of the atria. Up to 30% of patients with either type of atrial flutter develop AF late after a successful flutter ablation and may require further treatment; atrial flutter and AF often go together.

Key points – atrial flutter

- Ablation for typical atrial flutter is highly successful and low risk, and should be considered first-line treatment.
- The risk of systemic embolization in atrial flutter should be considered similar to that for atrial fibrillation (AF).
- Atypical atrial flutter usually includes right atrial flutter circling around regions of scarring, or left atrial flutter following ablation of AF.

Definition

Atrial fibrillation (AF) is an arrhythmia characterized by uncoordinated atrial activation with consequent deterioration of atrial mechanical function. The two key features of this condition are rapid atrial depolarization and an irregular ventricular response.

The rapidity of atrial depolarization (400–600 bpm) impairs effective atrial contractile function, increases stasis within the atrium and promotes the risk of systemic thromboembolism. Ventricular rates can vary widely from slow (30–40 bpm) to very rapid (occasionally about 200 bpm).

Epidemiology

Prevalence. AF is the most common sustained cardiac arrhythmia, affecting 1–2% of the general population. Its prevalence increases with age, hypertension, diabetes and the presence of structural cardiac disease. The condition can also occur without detectable disease (lone AF, see below). It has been estimated that at any one time 2.2 million Americans have paroxysmal or persistent AF (see Classification below).

Risk of developing AF. Of 4764 participants in the Framingham Heart Study monitored for a maximum of 10 years, 10% developed AF. Age, sex, body mass index, systolic blood pressure, treatment for hypertension, PR interval, clinically significant cardiac murmur and heart failure were all associated with the development of AF (Figure 8.1). In particular, risk of AF varied with age: more than 15% risk was recorded in only 1% of participants younger than 65 years, compared with 27% of those older than 65 years. In general, AF increases in prevalence with age (5–9% in the over-60s compared with 0.5–1.0% in the overall population), and is 1.5 times more common in women than men.

Healthcare costs. As discussed later in this chapter, AF carries a heavy economic burden because of its consequences – hemodynamic impairment, thromboembolic events and repeated hospital admissions. The total cost in the EU is estimated at €13.5 billion per year. AF costs approximately 1% of the healthcare budget in the UK and in France.

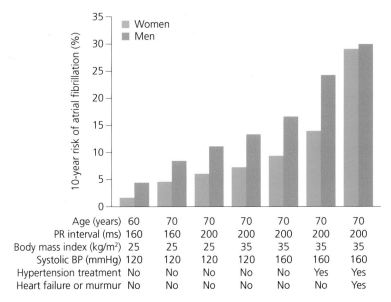

Figure 8.1 Risk factors associated with the development of atrial fibrillation in men and women over 10 years. Reprinted from *The Lancet* Schnabel RB et al. 2009;373:739–45, with permission from Elsevier.

Classification

AF is often viewed as a single entity but there are many different clinical patterns. Updated guidelines from the European Society of Cardiology (ESC) outline five main types of AF:

- **first diagnosed** – any patient who presents with AF for the first time irrespective of the duration of the arrhythmia or presence or severity of symptoms
- **paroxysmal** – recurrent AF (two or more episodes) that revert spontaneously to sinus rhythm , usually within 48 hours, although paroxysms may continue for up to 7 days
- **persistent** – recurrent AF that lasts longer than 7 days or needs to be reverted to sinus rhythm either pharmacologically or electrically
- **long-standing persistent** – continuous AF that lasts for 1 year or more while a rhythm control strategy is pursued
- **permanent** – the presence of AF is accepted by the patient (and physician), and restoration of sinus rhythm is not possible or is deemed impossible or not worthwhile.

Lone AF (AF in the absence of cardiovascular disease) is more common in younger patients (less than 60 years old). It occurs in 30–45% of paroxysmal cases and 20–25% of persistent cases. Lone AF is more benign in terms of thromboembolism and mortality and has a favorable prognosis. However, the prognosis worsens with the development of cardiac abnormalities, with a consequent increase in thromboembolism and mortality.

Causes

Causes of AF are shown in Table 8.1. In many cases, successful treatment of the underlying cause of acute AF eliminates the arrhythmia. AF secondary to a precipitating condition such as acute myocardial infarction (MI), cardiac surgery, myocarditis, hyperthyroidism or acute pulmonary disease should be considered separately (see below). In these circumstances, treatment of the underlying disorder concurrently with management of the episode of AF usually eliminates the arrhythmia. For example, abstinence after acute alcohol consumption often allows AF to revert back to sinus rhythm.

Pathophysiology

AF may present as a single episode (paroxysmal AF), but over time the frequency and duration increases, ultimately becoming sustained (see Classification above). In the early phase, AF is usually associated with persistent and repetitive firing of atrial foci within the pulmonary veins. Ectopic atrial tissue lies within the pulmonary veins where they enter the left atrium (see Figure 2.8b). Less frequently (15%), the foci arise in other venous structures such as the coronary sinus or superior vena cava. From here, intermittent and repetitive electrical firing spreads into the atrial tissue. This type of paroxysmal AF is occasionally termed focal AF.

Other factors implicated in the pathology of AF include mechanical issues that affect the atria and alterations in autonomic function. The pathological changes depend on the duration of fibrillation and the presence of any structural heart changes. An increase in the amount of fibrosis within the atria increases the risk of developing AF. Moderate to severe left atrial dilatation is also associated with an increased risk of AF. The exact role of these pathological changes in promoting AF is not known.

TABLE 8.1

Factors associated with an increased risk of atrial fibrillation (AF)

- Raised atrial pressure
- Systemic hypertension – often chronic over many years and particularly when LV hypertrophy is present
- Heart failure
- Atrial ischemia
- Atrial inflammation (e.g. postoperative acute pericarditis; after cardiac surgery up to 30% of patients may develop acute AF)
- Myocardial infarction
- Acute myocarditis
- Hypertrophic cardiomyopathy
- Pulmonary embolism
- Acute exacerbations of pulmonary diseases (e.g. asthma, COPD)
- Pheochromocytoma
- Severe electrolyte imbalance – severe hypokalemia (serum potassium < 2 mmol/L) or severe hyper/hypocalcemia; severe renal failure
- Surgery – particularly cardiac

- Acute infection; e.g. pneumonia
- Drugs (rarely) – intravenous adenosine can precipitate acute AF
- Alcohol (once called 'sailors' fibrillation')*
- Hyperthyroidism and hypothyroidism
- Endocrine abnormalities
- Autonomic, adrenergic or parasympathetic imbalance
- Electrocution
- Idiopathic AF
- Genetics
- Valvular heart disease (classically mitral stenosis and regurgitation)
- Coronary artery disease, particularly in the presence of impaired LV systolic function
- Some congenital heart diseases
- Obstructive sleep apnea
- Morbid obesity

*Quantity not well defined, but AF is associated with acute binges or chronic intake; also depends on individual susceptibility.
COPD, chronic obstructive pulmonary disease; LV, left ventricular.

In animal studies, the heart tends to remain in AF once the rhythm has been induced. If such AF is terminated quickly to sinus rhythm it is often difficult to reinitiate; the longer AF is present before termination the easier it becomes to reinitiate. Eventually, if left for long enough, it becomes increasingly difficult to obtain sinus rhythm, an observation paralleled in humans. Hence the term: 'atrial fibrillation begets atrial fibrillation'.

Once AF is sustained, the atria gradually dilate and fibrosis increases. Progressive atrial dilatation has been demonstrated by echocardiography in patients with AF, and can be either a cause or a consequence of persistent AF.

Consequences of atrial fibrillation

AF is not a benign condition. It is associated with a fivefold increase in stroke and double the mortality rate of similar aged 'normal' groups. AF also impairs left ventricular (LV) function, reduces exercise capacity and quality of life (QoL), and can result in recurrent hospitalization.

Loss of atrial contraction. Atrial filling can account for up to 30% of cardiac output, so loss of this function can result in a significant decrease in output. If there is structural heart disease (e.g. mitral stenosis, impaired diastolic ventricular filling, systemic hypertension, hypertrophic cardiomyopathy [HCM] or restrictive cardiomyopathies), loss of atrial systole combined with a variable heart rate (particularly if rapid) can precipitate catastrophic hemodynamic changes such as pulmonary edema, congestive cardiac failure or, rarely, complete hemodynamic collapse.

Systemic thromboembolism. Stroke and systemic arterial occlusion are generally attributed to embolism from the left atrium. Evidence that AF itself increases the risk of stroke is overwhelming: one-sixth of strokes occur in patients with AF. The rate of ischemic stroke among patients with non-rheumatic AF averages 5% per year. Rheumatic heart disease increases the risk of stroke significantly (in some reports up to 17-fold) compared with age-matched controls.

Irregularity of the ventricular response. The normal mechanisms that control the ventricular rate during sinus rhythm and prevent the heart from beating too quickly (e.g. during exercise) are lost in AF. Relatively minor exercise, like walking up stairs, may result in an inappropriately rapid ventricular response. The variation in heart rate may be severe (40–200 bpm) and often results in hemodynamic and symptomatic impairment.

Rarely, in patients with Wolff–Parkinson–White (WPW) syndrome (see Chapter 2) where the accessory pathway does not have the slowing capability of the atrioventricular (AV) node and can conduct rapidly, a potentially fatal outcome can occur. Conduction may occur predominantly over the pathway, allowing a very rapid ventricular response that degenerates to ventricular fibrillation (VF). Hence, drugs capable of blocking conduction through the AV node, such as digitalis and calcium-channel blockers, are contraindicated in patients with WPW syndrome, as these drugs do not block conduction over the accessory pathway.

Patients with HCM also fare badly during AF. Sudden death is well described in this group and the onset of AF is suspected to be one mechanism.

Inappropriate heart rate. It is increasingly recognized that a persistently elevated ventricular rate (130 bpm or faster in one study) can adversely affect LV function, causing a dilated cardiomyopathy, referred to as a tachycardiomyopathy. Adequate rate control can partially or even completely reverse this process. In many cases the ventricular rate is highly variable, often within a short time interval, which is known as the tachy–brady syndrome. It is often complex to manage, involving drugs that slow the rapid rates, which in turn can precipitate symptomatic bradycardias requiring electrical support in the form of a pacemaker.

Quality of life

Many studies have shown impaired QoL in patients with AF. However, it is difficult to determine whether AF is solely responsible for reduced wellbeing, as these patients often have comorbidities and are receiving multiple drug treatments. Long-term oral anticoagulant therapy, which involves frequent blood testing and multiple drug interactions, also affects the QoL of patients with AF.

Assessment

A highly systematic approach to assessment of AF is required:

- detect AF and confirm diagnosis
- identify the duration and type of AF
- assess symptom severity
- try to establish the cause
- assess complications and relevant comorbidities
- assess stroke risk
- assess risk of bleeding before anticoagulation
- organize further investigations.

Detect AF. Patients with AF are generally diagnosed once they are symptomatic; however, many have no overt symptoms and opportunistic screening for patients with an irregular pulse can facilitate detection. The SAFE study found that, in the primary care setting, opportunistic screening of patients aged 65 years and over, followed by an ECG when the pulse was irregular, was as effective as systematic screening for AF with an ECG. We would go further, and advise routine pulse checks for all patients over 50 years of age.

Physical examination, which should include pulse (rate and rhythm), blood pressure, jugular venous pressure, heart sounds, lungs and signs of peripheral edema, will highlight other features characteristic of AF (Table 8.2). A comprehensive history will ascertain any precipitating triggers such as exercise, alcohol or stress.

Confirm diagnosis. *If AF is suspected, an ECG should be performed immediately.* Even a single lead ECG is diagnostic, although a 12-lead ECG is always preferable. The key abnormality is a completely irregular, often rapid, ventricular response and loss of clear P waves, replaced by fibrillatory (or 'f') waves (Figure 8.2; also see Figure 2.8c). The ventricular response depends on the functional properties of the AV node, which reflects vagal and sympathetic tone and, in many cases, depends on the effects of drugs. While a slow regular heart rate (e.g. 40 bpm) may indicate the presence of heart block, a slow but variable heart rate indicates a slow ventricular response during AF, and is often drug related. Very rapid ventricular rates (over 200 bpm) associated with a wide QRS complex may indicate the presence of an accessory pathway, or bundle branch block.

TABLE 8.2

Features to look for during physical examination

- Irregular pulse
- Irregular jugular venous pulsations
- Associated heart failure
- Associated myocardial abnormalities (e.g. HCM – jerky carotid pulse and systolic murmur)
- Associated valvular heart disease – mitral regurgitation or stenosis; mitral valve prolapse

HCM, hypertrophic cardiomyopathy.

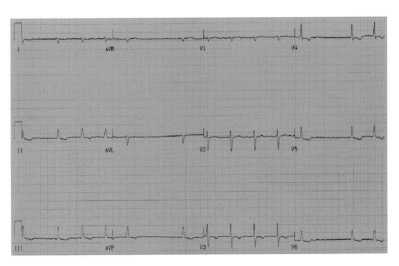

Figure 8.2 A 12-lead ECG of atrial fibrillation. There are no discernable P waves on the baseline and the QRS response is completely irregular.

Identify the duration and type of AF. The duration of a first-detected episode of AF, either symptomatic or self-limiting, is likely to be uncertain, and the clinician must recognize the likelihood of previous undetected episodes. However, it is important to determine the type of AF (see Classification, page 73), because it determines overall management: a first episode requires assessment for future drug therapy and anticoagulation

79

but a single self-terminating episode may not require intervention; persistent AF requires rhythm control; and permanent AF requires rate control. Deciding whether to accept AF, pursue anticoagulation and control the ventricular response, or to restore and maintain sinus rhythm by cardioversion and/or other strategies is not always straightforward. A detailed history is helpful in determining whether AF is paroxysmal or persistent.

Assess symptom severity. The clinical presentation of AF can be highly variable; patients may be asymptomatic or may present with a range of symptoms (Table 8.3). Clearly, the severity of symptoms will determine both the immediate and long-term management strategies (rate control or rhythm control, see pages 90–3). ESC guidelines suggest using the European Heart Rhythm Association (EHRA) symptom score as a means of assessing those symptoms that are attributable only to AF and reverse

TABLE 8.3

Clinical presentations of atrial fibrillation

Symptom	Pathophysiological cause
Palpitations	Change in ventricular rate and rhythm
Shortness of breath or chest pains	Loss of functional cardiac capacity
Fatigue	Loss of functional cardiac capacity
Heart failure	Deterioration in left ventricular systolic function (tachycardiomyopathy due to persistently fast ventricular rates) or AF in the presence of structural heart disease
Presyncope and syncope	Slow ventricular rates: less commonly very rapid rates
Thromboembolism	Stroke (usually) Renal or bowel (rarely)

Polyuria (rarely)*

*Comes on 20–30 minutes after the onset of the arrhythmia and is associated only with paroxysmal AF rather than persistent or permanent AF.

TABLE 8.4

EHRA score for atrial fibrillation-related symptoms

EHRA	Symptom severity
I	No symptoms
II	Mild symptoms: normal daily activity not affected
III	Severe symptoms: normal daily activity affected
IV	Disabling symptoms: normal daily activity discontinued

EHRA, European Heart Rhythm Association.

or reduce when sinus rhythm is restored or with effective rate control (Table 8.4)

Try to establish the cause (see Table 8.1). It may be possible to identify specific precipitants in some patients (e.g. chest infection, excessive alcohol). Enquiry should also be made for symptoms of thyrotoxicosis.

Assess complications and relevant comorbidities such as previous transient ischemic attacks (TIAs)/cerebral vascular accident, systemic hypertension, diabetes mellitus, ischemic heart disease and previous MI. A history of undiagnosed dyspepsia or gastrointestinal bleeding may be relevant to the use of anticoagulation therapy. Renal and hepatic function should also be assessed.

Assess stroke risk. AF is a major cause of embolic stroke. The original $CHADS_2$ score is a simple and easy-to-remember risk assessment scheme particularly suited to use by primary care practitioners and non-specialists. Points are allocated as follows:
- Congestive heart failure (1)
- Hypertension, or treated hypertension (1)
- Age > 75 years (1)
- Diabetes mellitus (1)
- (previous) Stroke or TIA (2).

This has now been refined to include scoring for specific age categories, the presence of vascular disease and female sex, all important risk factors as nearly half of AF-associated strokes occur in patients over 75 years of age, and AF is the most frequent cause of disabling stroke in elderly women. Known as CHA_2DS_2VASc, the new scoring system provides a more detailed assessment of stroke risk. Points are allocated as follows:

- Congestive heart failure/LV dysfunction (1)
- Hypertension, or treated hypertension (1)
- Age > 75 years (2)
- Diabetes mellitus (1)
- Stroke/TIA/thromboembolism (2)
- Vascular disease (1)
- Age 65–74 years (1)
- Sex (female) (1).

The higher the total score the greater the risk of stroke (Table 8.5) and thus the level of anticoagulation therapy required.

Risk of bleeding must be assessed before anticoagulation therapy is started. There are three recognized scoring systems to assess bleeding risk: $HEMORR_2HAGES$ (Hepatic or renal disease, Ethanol abuse, Malignancy,

TABLE 8.5

Annual stroke risk calculated from the CHA_2DS_2VASc* score

CHA_2DS_2VASc	Patients (n=7329)	Stroke risk (%/year)
0	1	0
1	422	1.3
2	1230	2.2
3	1730	3.2
4	1718	4.0
5	1159	6.7
6	679	9.8
7	294	9.6
8	82	6.7
9	14	15.2

*C, congestive heart failure; H, hypertension; A, age (> 75 years); D, diabetes; S, (prior) stroke (TIA/thromboembolism); V, vascular heart disease; A, age (65–74 years); S, sex (female).

Older age, Reduced platelet count or function, Re-bleeding, Hypertension, Anemia, Genetic factors, Excessive fall risk and Stroke), ATRIA (Anticoagulation and Risk factors In Atrial fibrillation) and HAS-BLED (Hypertension, Abnormal renal/liver function, Stroke, Bleeding history or predisposition, Labile international normalized ratio, Elderly and Drugs/alcohol). The HAS-BLED scoring system estimates the risk of major bleeding for patients on anticoagulant medication (Table 8.6). It can be used in conjunction with the CHA_2DS_2VASc score (as described above) to determine if anticoagulation is in the best interest of the patient. For example, older people are at increased risk for anticoagulant-related bleeding and are therefore less likely to be treated with oral anticoagulation, even in situations for which efficacy is proven. A HAS-BLED score of 3 or higher is considered 'high risk', and such patients should be reviewed regularly.

Organize other investigations

Thyroid function tests are mandatory.

Transthoracic echocardiography can provide useful information to guide clinical decision making. It is valuable for defining valvular or structural heart disease associated with AF, but it cannot exclude thrombus in the left atrial appendage (LAA). Some studies have shown that moderate-to-severe LV dysfunction is an independent echocardiographic predictor of stroke.

In North America, an echocardiogram would usually be obtained during the initial work-up of AF. In the UK, the National Institute for Health and Clinical Excellence (NICE) recommends transthoracic echocardiography in AF patients:

- for whom a baseline echocardiogram is important for long-term management (e.g. younger patients)
- for whom a rhythm control strategy is being considered (pharmacological or electrical cardioversion)
- with a high risk of underlying heart disease that will influence subsequent management (echocardiography will detect structural defects such as valvular heart disease or cardiomyopathy)
- who require refinement of clinical risk stratification for antithrombotic therapy.

Transesophageal echocardiography is a far more sensitive and specific imaging technique for detection of thrombus within the left atrium and

TABLE 8.6

The HASBLED scoring system for assessment of major bleeding* risk with anticoagulation

	Clinical characteristic	Score
H	Hypertension (uncontrolled, > 160 mmHg systolic)	1
A	Abnormal renal function (dialysis; transplant; serum Cr > 2.6 mg/dL or > 200 µmol/L)	1
	Abnormal liver function (cirrhosis; bilirubin > 2 x normal; AST/ALT/AP > 3 x normal)	1
S	Stroke history	1
B	Bleeding history or predisposition to bleeding	1
L	Labile INRs (unstable/high INRs, < 60% time in therapeutic range)	1
E	Elderly (age > 75 years)	1
D	Drugs usage predisposing to bleeding (e.g. antiplatelet therapy, NSAIDs)	1
	or	
	Alcohol usage history	1
		Maximum score 9

*Major bleeding was defined in the HAS-BLED study as intracranial (requiring hospitalization), hemoglobin decrease > 2 g/L and/or transfusion.
ALT, alanine aminotransferase; AP, alkaline phosphatase; AST, aspartate aminotransferase; Cr, creatinine; INR, international normalized ratio; NSAID, non-steroidal anti-inflammatory drug. Adapted from Pisters R et al. 2010.

LAA and is the imaging modality of choice when a left atrial thrombus is clinically suspected.

A chest radiograph may also be useful, particularly when determining management.

An exercise stress test is useful if coronary ischemia is suspected. In patients unable to exercise, dobutamine stress echo or nuclear imaging should be used.

24-hour monitoring. If episodes are frequent, a 24-hour Holter monitor may help to establish the diagnosis and provide a permanent ECG record of the dysrrhythmia (see page 42). If episodes are infrequent, then an event recorder, which allows the patient to transmit the ECG to a recording facility when the arrhythmia occurs, may be more useful.

A Holter monitor is useful to determine the ventricular rate during AF, which helps to assess the effectiveness of drug therapy. Many patients with symptomatic AF also have asymptomatic AF and a Holter gives an idea of AF burden.

Electrophysiological studies are only helpful if an accessory pathway or a different arrhythmia is suspected.

Management

The management of patients with AF involves both the arrhythmia itself and the prevention of thromboembolism by anticoagulation (see pages 104–7). Treatment will depend upon where and how the patient presents.

Management in general practice. AF is the most common arrhythmia encountered in primary care, and is often diagnosed as an incidental finding during a routine medical check. Table 8.7 provides an overview of management in this setting, according to the clinical presentation.

If AF is found incidentally or on the first presentation, and the duration is not known for certain (it is often difficult to be certain of the duration), stroke risk should be assessed (see page 81–2) and anticoagulation initiated with a vitamin K antagonist (VKA) or similar agents for all patients except those with a CHA_2DS_2Vasc score of 0 (for anticoagulation regimens see Table 8.11), along with rate control therapy.

If the patient's symptoms are stable then anticoagulation and rate control can be considered in the primary care setting, unless other clinical factors warrant referral (e.g. frail, non-compliant, concurrent dementia, other severe debilitating illness). Beta-blockers are effective for rate control, and short-acting beta-blockers (e.g. metoprolol) may be particularly helpful when initiating treatment. If there is no past history of heart failure or remote MI, then calcium antagonists (diltiazem or verapamil) can also be helpful, but be wary of combining calcium antagonists and beta-blockers, as significant bradycardia can be induced; otherwise, consider digoxin if indicated.

Renal function, fasting blood sugar and thyroid function should be checked, and underlying causes excluded (e.g. thyroid disease, heart

TABLE 8.7

Management in general practice

Presentation	Action
Complete hemodynamic collapse (rare in AF)	CPR
	Call ambulance
	Immediate transfer to hospital
Recent history of chest pain and palpitations; irregularly irregular pulse	ECG*, admit to hospital
Highly symptomatic (e.g. severe palpitations, diaphoretic, breathless); rapid, irregularly irregular pulse; hemodynamically stable	ECG*, admit to hospital
Persistent palpitations for > 24 hours; irregularly irregular pulse	ECG*; if AF is confirmed, admit to hospital for possible rate control and anticoagulation
Stable symptoms (e.g. SOB, progressive ankle edema, tiredness or lack of energy); irregularly irregular pulse	ECG*
	Consider stroke and hemorrhagic risk (with treatment)
	Consider immediate anticoagulation, rate control and further investigation (see text)

*12-lead ECG is always preferable.
CPR, cardiopulmonary resuscitation; SOB, shortness of breath.

disease). A chest X-ray and thoracic echocardiography can help with clinical decision making (see pages 83–4).

Many episodes of AF terminate spontaneously within the first hours or days, but if patients remain symptomatic despite adequate rate control cardiologic referral is recommended, as there are different treatment modalities depending upon whether the AF is paroxysmal, persistent or permanent (see Treatment by type of AF below).

The decision to pursue rhythm control must be tailored to the individual patient. The clinician should assess how permanent AF is likely to affect the patient in the future and how successful rhythm control is expected to be, taking into account symptom severity, age and activity levels. Advice on lifestyle modification should include support for alcohol reduction/ abstinence and stopping smoking, alongside aggressive management of systemic hypertension and diabetes.

Acute hospital management. If the patient presents with hemodynamic collapse, then emergency DC cardioversion is essential. For acute ventricular rate control, intravenous beta-blockers or amiodarone (300 mg bolus) should be administered.

If the AF is *definitely* known to be of short duration, particularly for less than 24 hours, intravenous chemical cardioversion with flecainide or ibutilide (USA) should be considered, provided it is not contraindicated (good LV function, no past history of ischemic heart disease/MI etc.). If contraindicated, intravenous amiodarone (300 mg bolus over 30 minutes) should be administered instead. Once any underlying causes (thyroid disease, other heart conditions, hypertension, acute alcohol abuse) have been excluded, if one drug is unsuccessful and the AF has *definitely* been present for less than 24 hours, then external DC cardioversion should be considered. If one drug is unsuccessful, the patient remains highly symptomatic and there is doubt about whether the AF has lasted for 24 hours or longer, a transesophageal-guided echocardiocardiogram (TOE) should be considered to exclude a thrombus within the left atrium/appendage.

When the history suggests that AF may have been ongoing for over 48 hours, or if it is difficult to be certain, then oral anticoagulation and drug-based rate control should be initiated in uncompromised patients, with a view to an elective cardioversion in 4–8 weeks.

The need for long-term antiarrhythmic medication should be assessed; for example, if AF is the first presentation of mitral valve disease then both long-term antiarrhythmic drugs and anticoagulation are required.

Treatment by type of atrial fibrillation

As discussed in the Classification section (see page 73), AF can progress from paroxysmal to persistent or permanent forms, and is at times symptomatic. The type of AF and severity of symptoms will determine the nature of the treatment (Figure 8.3).

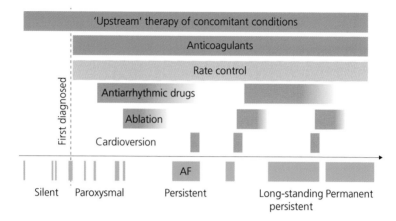

Figure 8.3 The type of atrial fibrillation (AF) will determine the nature of the treatment. The natural course of AF is shown along the baseline against a background of sinus rhythm. Typical therapeutic measures to improve symptoms and cardiovascular outcomes are shown in the boxes above in relation to the type of AF. Reprinted from Camm AJ et al. 2010 ESC Guidelines, by permission of the European Society of Cardiology.

Management of paroxysmal AF. Patients who have infrequent (once or twice per year) self-limiting episodes of paroxysmal AF and no structural heart disease do not usually require antiarrhythmic treatment (Figure 8.4). The decision to anticoagulate should be individualized for each patient and will depend on a balance between their intrinsic risk of thromboembolism (CHA$_2$DS$_2$VASc score) and the risk of bleeding (see pages 81–3).

Rate control treatment becomes necessary when symptoms become intrusive (e.g. symptomatic palpitations, hypotension, myocardial ischemia or heart failure) or episodes become more frequent. The initial selection of antiarrhythmic drugs should be based on safety (see pages 93–4).

Management of persistent AF. Once the diagnosis has been confirmed, anticoagulation and rate control should be provided as needed. If DC cardioversion is being considered then anticoagulation with either warfarin or a newer oral anticoagulant (dabigatran, apixaban, rivaroxaban) should be considered. Rate control agents include beta-blockers (particularly if LV function is impaired), calcium antagonists (to be avoided in patients with poor LV function) and digoxin (poor at rate

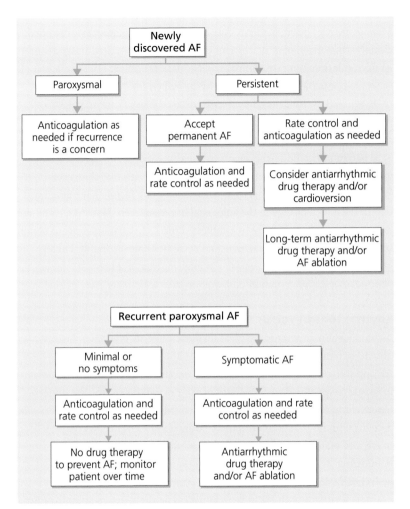

Figure 8.4 Management of patients with newly discovered paroxysmal or persistent atrial fibrillation (AF) and recurrent paroxysmal AF. HF, heart failure.

control during exercise). The long-term side effects of drugs such as amiodarone must be taken into account if considering their use purely for rate control.

Cardiologic referral is recommended to assess long-term management, i.e. whether rhythm control with cardioversion or ablation is appropriate or if rate control therapy should be continued, leaving the patient in long-standing persistent or permanent AF (see Figure 8.4).

Management of permanent AF. Any underlying causes must be identified, along with management of any comorbidites and associated heart disease. Anticoagulation and rate control are the main treatment goals, unless it is deemed possible to restore sinus rhythm when the AF category is re-designated as 'long-standing persistent' (see Classification, page 73). Anticoagulation needs to find the balance between reducing the stroke rate and hemorrhagic complications.

If patients become asymptomatic or mildly symptomatic they can be maintained on rate control therapy for years, although they may need infrequent monitoring to ascertain whether any risk factors have developed that necessitate a change in the anticoagulation regimen. However, it should be noted that once AF has been established for 2–3 years, attempts to obtain sinus rhythm are more challenging and more often unsuccessful. Highly symptomatic patients may require a change in drug or a non-pharmacological intervention (ablation or pace and ablate – see below).

Rhythm control versus rate control

Although sinus rhythm is the ideal, in some patients it is difficult to obtain/maintain and sometimes it may be appropriate to accept long-term AF and just control the ventricular rate. Several large multicenter studies have addressed this issue. A variety of factors will determine the preferred treatment approach in each individual patient. For example, a 70-year-old patient, with no (or mild) symptoms and a good QoL may be better left in AF and managed with anticoagulation/rate control therapy and monitoring. Clinical assessment of the best strategy should be reviewed periodically depending on the patient's symptoms. In some cases, for example a patient with slight breathlessness or slight fatigue that may or may not be due to AF, an attempt at cardioversion may be appropriate to see if the patient feels any different. Sometimes a patient may not realize how much better they can feel until they experience normal sinus rhythm. However, once AF has been established for more than 3 years, attempts to obtain sinus rhythm are generally ineffective. The final decision will depend on the balance between the risks and side effects of treatment and the effects of AF.

Optimal rate control has previously aimed at a resting heart rate of 60–80 bpm and 90–115 bpm during moderate exercise. However, recent trial results (RACE II) did not identify a benefit of strict rate control over lenient rate control (< 110 bpm at rest), suggesting that lenient rate control, in patients without severe symptoms at least, is a reasonable strategy to adopt.

Restoration of sinus rhythm is the aim in many patients with persistent AF (Figure 8.5). In general, this is an elective procedure but the need for cardioversion may be immediate if the arrhythmia is the main factor responsible for acute heart failure or severe hypotension. Cardioversion can be achieved by means of drugs or electrical shocks (see Chapter 5).

Pharmacological cardioversion appears to be most effective when initiated early, preferably within 24 hours of AF onset, although it may be effective within 7 days. Most patients have paroxysmal AF, a first-documented episode of AF or an unknown pattern of AF at the time of treatment. A large proportion of patients with recent-onset AF experience spontaneous cardioversion within 24–48 hours. This is less likely to occur when AF has persisted for more than 7 days. For patients who present with AF incidentally or in whom symptoms are mild, starting a beta-

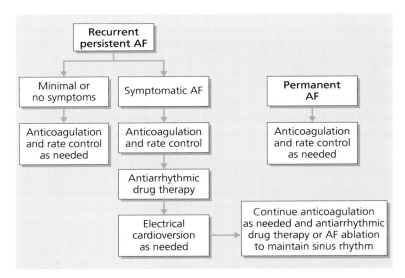

Figure 8.5 Management of patients with recurrent persistent or permanent atrial fibrillation (AF). Drug therapy may be initiated before cardioversion to reduce the likelihood of early recurrence of AF.

blocker in an outpatient setting may be adequate pending further assessment. The major concern when considering the termination of AF is the potential for serious adverse effects, including *torsades de pointes* (rare) and sinus node dysfunction (which is more usual in the elderly).

Generally, when AF has been established for more than 48 hours, anticoagulation should be given and the patient asked to return for elective cardioversion in about 6 weeks.

In acute cases, ECG monitoring during pharmacological conversion is mandatory. If LV function is preserved, intravenous flecainide or ibutilide (USA) is useful. If LV function is impaired or poor, or suspected to be so (previous MI, heart failure, long-standing hypertension), then intravenous amiodarone is preferable, or intravenous digoxin may be useful. Beta-blockers should be avoided in the presence of acute heart failure. If it is deemed clinically important to obtain sinus rhythm (e.g. AF in the presence of mitral stenosis) amiodarone is usually the most successful agent.

Direct-current (DC) cardioversion. In selected cases the primary success rate is 85–90%.

Contraindications. There are few direct contraindications to DC cardioversion – these are mainly related to anesthetic risk or the presence of a known intracardiac thrombus or mass – and it is reasonable to make at least one attempt to restore sinus rhythm in a patient with persistent AF. Asymptomatic AF in patients over 75 years of age (i.e. discovered on routine examination) may be best treated medically, especially if the patient has long-standing hypertension. The potential toxicity of antiarrhythmic drugs may outweigh the benefit of restoring sinus rhythm.

Maintenance of sinus rhythm with drugs is relevant in patients with paroxysmal or persistent AF. If the decision is made to cardiovert and maintain sinus rhythm, most patients should be considered for anticoagulation and prophylactic drug therapy to prevent recurrence of AF (Figure 8.6). Drugs with few side effects should be used first, accepting that many of the most effective agents have the most concerning side-effect profile. Long-term antiarrhythmic medication is likely, as the risk of relapse will be high, especially in elderly patients; however, some patients may require only 6–12 months of prophylactic drug therapy.

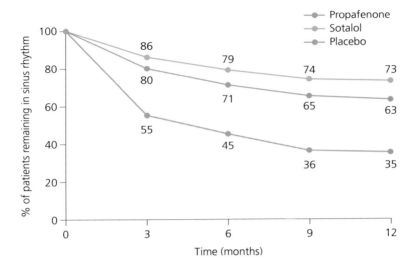

Figure 8.6 Kaplan–Meier estimates of the percentage of patients remaining in sinus rhythm during follow-up, after conversion of recurrent symptomatic atrial fibrillation. After 1 year of follow-up, the proportion of patients remaining in sinus rhythm was comparable between propafenone (63%) and sotalol (73%) and superior to placebo (35%; p=0.001 versus both drugs). Reprinted from Bellandi F et al. *Am J Cardiol* 2001;88:640–5, with permission from Elsevier.

Patients with permanent AF in whom sinus rhythm cannot be obtained or maintained should be treated for ventricular rate control and anticoagulation. If there is a suspicion that LV dysfunction may be due to unsatisfactory rate control, and drugs are not effectively stabilizing the rate, an 'ablate and pace' strategy should be considered (see pages 102–3).

Pharmacological treatment

Drug therapy for ventricular rate control. Before any antiarrhythmic agent is administered, reversible cardiovascular and non-cardiovascular precipitants of AF should be addressed. Several agents that slow conduction in the AV node can be effective for ventricular rate control depending on the clinical setting (Table 8.8).

Generic side effects. All drugs have potential side effects, but antiarrhythmic therapy in general has two generic effects – negative

TABLE 8.8

Drugs that slow conduction in the atrioventricular node

Acute AF

Beta-blockers	Esmolol (i.v. only)	0.5 mg/kg over 1 min
	Metoprolol	2.5–5 mg i.v. bolus
Calcium-channel blockers	Diltiazem	0.25 mg/kg over 2 mins
	Verapamil	0.075–0.15 mg/kg over 2 mins

Chronic AF

Beta-blockers	Metoprolol	25–100 mg twice daily
	Bisoprolol	2.5–10 mg/day
Calcium-channel blockers	Diltiazem	120–360 mg/day slow release
	Verapamil	120–360 mg/day
	Digoxin	0.125–0.375 mg/day

inotropism and proarrhythmia – which must be borne in mind when selecting initial drugs (see Chapter 5). As the disease progresses a drug that was initially safe may become proarrhythmic or negatively inotropic if, for example, coronary artery disease (CAD) or heart failure develops. Additional medication for other conditions may increase the risk of proarrhythmia. Thus, the patient should be alerted to the potential significance of symptoms such as syncope, angina pectoris and dyspnea, and warned about the use of non-cardiac drugs that can prolong the QT interval. A useful source of information is www.azcert.org. Patients must be warned that syncope or presyncope are important symptoms and that they should seek medical advice urgently. Progressive breathlessness may be an indication of worsening heart failure.

Antiarrhythmic drugs

Amiodarone reduces the frequency of episodes but must be used carefully in light of its side effects, including thyroid dysfunction, which can take years to manifest, and requires careful monitoring. The lowest effective dose should be used, often 200 mg/day. Larger doses result in an increased incidence of side effects, such as liver dysfunction, hyper- or hypothyroidism, pulmonary fibrosis, sun sensitivity and visual disturbances. Amiodarone potentiates the effects of warfarin, so the warfarin dose should be reduced when initiating amiodarone therapy.

Dronedarone is indicated for the treatment of AF in patients whose hearts have either returned to normal rhythm or who undergo drug therapy or electric shock treatment to maintain normal rhythm. Although only recently approved in 2009, a report in 2011 investigating the use of dronedarone in patients with permanent AF (PALLAS) was stopped early because of a two-fold increase in death, stroke and hospitalization for heart failure in patients receiving dronedarone compared with those taking a placebo. As patients with paroxysmal AF may develop persistent AF, there has been concern that dronedarone may continue to be used in all patients with AF regardless of type. Furthermore, concerns of liver toxicity, and risks associated with administration of dronedarone in patients with renal failure and heart failure, have significantly limited clinical use of the drug.

Digoxin remains a useful drug as an adjunct to beta-blockers and amiodarone, particularly for rate control in patients with heart failure. However, it has its limitations: while digoxin controls ventricular rate at rest, it is less effective during exercise. It is also contraindicated in patients with paroxysmal AF, as it can increase the frequency of AF episodes.

Flecainide can be given orally or intravenously. The usual oral dose is 100–200 mg/day in divided doses. It should be avoided if creatinine clearance is less than 50 mg/mL, and in patients with LV hypertrophy and impaired LV function (< 40% ejection fraction) and CAD. The dose should be reduced or the drug discontinued if the QRS width increases by more than 25%. Flecainide should be used with care if conduction system disease is present, and if the patient has new symptoms of syncope the drug should be stopped immediately.

Propafenone is given orally, usually at a dose of 150–300 mg three times a day. It should be avoided in patients with CAD and reduced ejection fraction, and used with caution in patients with reduced renal function or conduction disease.

Sotalol is given orally at a dose of 80–160 mg twice daily. It prolongs the QT interval, so the dose should be reduced or the drug discontinued if the QTc is greater than 500 ms. Sotalol should be avoided in patients with heart failure, depressed LV function and impaired renal function (creatinine clearance < 50mL/min). It should not be used with other QT-prolonging drugs. It is a useful initial drug in male patients with paroxysmal AF and normal hearts.

Choice of antiarrhythmic drug. Prophylactic drug treatment is seldom indicated in a first episode of AF unless there are extenuating circumstances like a severely debilitating episode. Drug therapy can also be avoided in patients with infrequent well-tolerated paroxysmal AF. Similarly, when recurrences are infrequent and tolerated, a patient experiencing breakthrough arrhythmias may not require a change in antiarrhythmic drug therapy. When treatment with a single drug fails, combinations of antiarrhythmic drugs may be tried. Useful combinations include a beta-blocker and amiodarone, and, if LV function is normal, a beta-blocker and an agent like flecainide. Figure 8.7 shows the choice of antiarrhythmic drug treatment in patients with or without heart disease.

Without heart disease. For individuals with no, or minimal, structural heart disease, flecainide, propafenone, sotalol, dronedarone or a selective beta-blocker such as metoprolol or bisoprolol are useful. They are generally well tolerated and have little extracardiac toxicity. Many of these drugs (flecainide, propafenone, amiodarone, dronedarone) have potentially serious side effects and should only be started by a cardiologist.

Exercise-induced AF. Beta-blockers can be effective in exercise-induced AF, but few patients have a single specific inciting cause for all episodes of AF, and the majority will not maintain sinus rhythm without antiarrhythmic drug treatment.

Lone AF and vagally mediated AF. In patients with lone AF, a beta-blocker may be tried first, but flecainide, propafenone and sotalol are particularly effective. Dofetilide is recommended as alternative therapy, but other therapies should be considered before initiating treatment with amiodarone because of its significant long-term side effects.

Adrenergically mediated AF. First-line treatment is with beta-blockers, followed by sotalol. Amiodarone can be used, but should be chosen later in the sequence of drug therapy because of its potential toxicity.

Heart failure. Patients with congestive heart failure or impaired LV systolic function are prone to both the proarrhythmic and negative inotropic effects of antiarrhythmic drugs (see Chapter 5). Flecainide and propafenone are contraindicated. Randomized trials have demonstrated the safety of

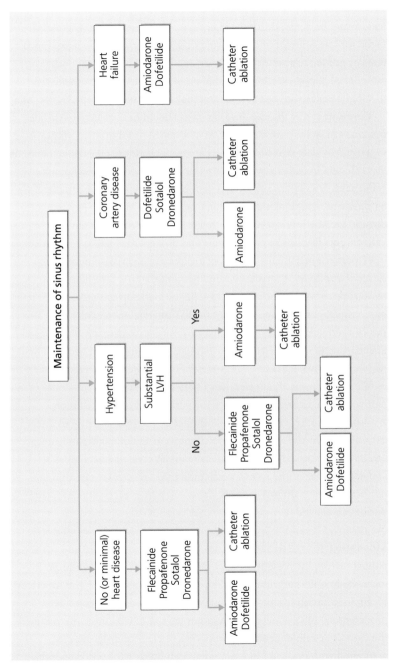

Figure 8.7 Choice of antiarrhythmic drug for the treatment of atrial fibrillation.

amiodarone or dofetilide for the maintenance of sinus rhythm. Digoxin is useful for rate control but does not alter the frequency of AF in paroxysmal cases or prevent relapse after cardioversion. Digoxin is also not effective at rate control during exercise. The addition of a beta-blocker to amiodarone is useful in patients with heart failure but may lead to symptomatic bradycardia.

Coronary artery disease. Beta-blockers should be considered first-line treatment in stable patients with CAD, although proof of their efficacy is supported by only two studies, and data on their efficacy for maintenance of sinus rhythm in patients with persistent AF after cardioversion are not convincing. Sotalol has substantial beta-blocking activity and can therefore be chosen as the initial antiarrhythmic agent in patients with ischemic heart disease, because it is associated with less long-term toxicity than amiodarone. Flecainide, propafenone and dronedarone are to be avoided.

Hypertension. Patients with LVH are at increased risk of developing *torsades de pointes.* Propafenone and flecainide with a beta-blocker are reasonable choices in the absence of CAD or marked ventricular hypertrophy. Amiodarone prolongs the QT interval but carries a very low risk of ventricular proarrhythmia. Its extracardiac toxicity profile relegates amiodarone to second-line therapy in these individuals but it becomes first-line therapy when marked LVH is present (avoid flecainide/propafenone).

WPW syndrome. Radiofrequency ablation (RFA) of the accessory pathway is the treatment of choice for patients with pre-excitation syndromes and AF, and all patients should be referred urgently to a cardiologist for assessment. In rare circumstances, antiarrhythmic drugs can be used, although digoxin and calcium-channel blockers must be avoided because of the risk of accelerating the ventricular rate during AF. Beta-blockers do not decrease conduction over accessory pathways during pre-excited periods of AF.

Monitoring of drug treatment varies with the agent involved and with patient factors. At present, data on the upper limits of drug-induced increases in QRS duration or QT interval are not available. The American Heart Association recommends that with class 1c drugs (flecainide, propafenone) QRS widening should not exceed 150% of the pretreatment duration. The rate-dependency properties of class 1c drugs may be associated with marked QRS widening with increased heart rates, which may be associated with proarrhythmia.

For class 1a and class 3 drugs, with the possible exception of amiodarone, the corrected QT interval in sinus rhythm should remain below 520 ms. Plasma potassium and magnesium levels and renal function should be checked periodically during follow-up. Clinical state and LV function should be reassessed in selected patients, especially if clinical heart failure develops during treatment of AF.

Non-pharmacological treatment

Catheter ablation. The principles and rationale for pulmonary vein isolation (PVI) for paroxysmal AF are:

- 75–96% of patients with paroxysmal AF have pulmonary vein foci that trigger AF
- electrical disconnection of the pulmonary vein from the body of the left atrium prevents AF in 70–80% of patients
- ostial or periostial ablation is safer than ablation within the vein, reducing the risk of pulmonary vein stenosis
- in some cases a complex combination of ablation within the atria and pulmonary vein isolation is required.

Transesophageal echocardiography prior to ablation is recommended. Detection of thrombus in the left atrium is a contraindication to elective ablation.

The ablation procedure is discussed in Chapter 5. In AF, point-by-point ablation lesions electrically isolate the pulmonary veins from the left atrium proper (Figure 8.8). Non-fluoroscopic three-dimensional mapping systems provide an anatomic map while the catheter is in the heart, helping the operator to navigate the complex patient-specific anatomy involved in the procedure (Figure 8.9).

Balloon technology can also be used to isolate the pulmonary veins (Figure 8.10). Magnetic and robotic methods of ablation have also been developed. Intracardiac echocardiography can further assist the operator during ablation of AF.

The use of non-fluoroscopic mapping, intracardiac echocardiography and robotic systems has been associated with a reduction in fluoroscopy duration, hence reducing the operator's exposure to radiation during long procedures; in fact, recent reports have demonstrated that AF ablation performed with these systems can be completed without the need for any fluoroscopy.

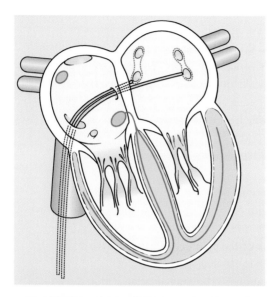

Figure 8.8 Transseptal puncture approach to catheter ablation for the treatment of atrial fibrillation, showing electrical isolation of the pulmonary veins.

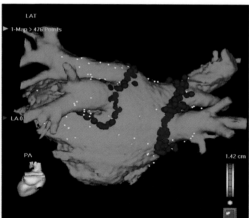

Figure 8.9 Three-dimensional electroanatomic mapping system. The ablation lesions, represented as red dots, are placed in a point-by-point fashion to electrically isolate the pulmonary veins.

A recent Expert Consensus Statement by seven international cardiac organizations has published formal indications for catheter ablation with level-of-evidence designations for each indication (Table 8.9). These stratify patients by type of AF and whether the procedure is being performed before or after a trial of one or more antiarrhythmic drugs. ESC guidelines state that catheter ablation is more effective than long-term antiarrhythmic therapy and should be considered first-line treatment in selected patients with paroxysmal AF.

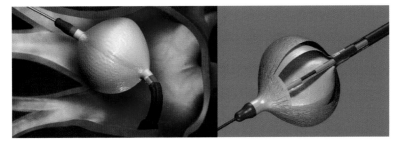

Figure 8.10 Balloon ablation catheters, which electrically isolate the pulmonary veins rapidly, are under evaluation in clinical trials in the USA. Images reproduced courtesy of Medtronic.

TABLE 8.9

Indications for catheter ablation of atrial fibrillation

	Indication	Class	Level of evidence
Symptomatic AF, refractory or intolerant to at least one class 1 or 3 antiarrhythmic medication			
Paroxysmal	Recommended*	I	A
Persistent	Reasonable	IIa	B
Long-standing persistent	May be considered	IIb	B
Symptomatic AF prior to initiation of antiarrhythmic drug therapy with a class 1 or 3 antiarrhythmic agent			
Paroxysmal	Reasonable	IIa	B
Persistent	May be considered	IIb	C
Long-standing persistent	May be considered	IIb	C

*Only when performed by an appropriately trained electrophysiologist in an experienced center.
Class I, the benefits markedly exceed the risks and should be performed; Class IIa, the benefits exceed the risks and it is reasonable to perform the procedure; Class IIb, the benefits are greater or equal to the risks and the procedure may be considered.
Evidence levels: A, data derived from multiple randomized clinical trials or meta-analyses; B, data derived from a single randomized trial or non-randomized studies; C, primary source of recommendation was consensus opinion/clinical experience, case studies or standard of care.
Source: 2012 HRS/EHRA/ECAS Expert Consensus Statement on Catheter and Surgical Ablation of Atrial Fibrillation: Recommendations for Patient Selection, Procedural Techniques, Patient Management and Follow-up, Definitions, Endpoints, and Research Trial Design.

Additional variables to consider when assessing whether a patient is a suitable candidate for ablation include the presence of concomitant heart disease, obesity/sleep apnea, left atrial size and the duration of time a patient has been in continuous AF. Patient preference (e.g. for a non-pharmacological approach) is also important. While some centers are now successfully eliminating AF with a low complication rate in up to 80–90% of cases of paroxysmal AF using PVI, patients should be counseled about the small but serious risks involved (Table 8.10).

The technique is more complex and demanding in patients with persistent AF because the structure and function of the atria change with time in a manner that favors perpetuation of the arrhythmia. Even in the best-case scenario a 50% relapse rate within 12 months remains and 50% of patients require a repeat procedure. The results following a second procedure are encouraging. This is an increasingly successful technique, but it does not rid patients of the need to take warfarin long term; this will change as success rates improve.

Pacemakers. Many types of atrial pacing have been explored. None has provided a suitable level of success to be recommended as first-line treatment, but some highly selected patients do benefit. Pacemakers are discussed in greater detail in Chapter 11.

'Ablate and pace' for ventricular rate control. AV nodal ablation and implantation of a permanent pacemaker ('ablate and pace') can improve QoL in patients with symptoms related to a rapid ventricular rate during AF that cannot be adequately controlled with antiarrhythmic medications. AV nodal ablation is particularly useful when an excessive ventricular rate induces tachycardiomyopathy. The technique is straightforward with virtually no risk of thromboembolism, and patients may not require sedation.

The ablate and pace option is highly successful at abolishing palpitations due to unacceptable ventricular rates. Once in place, the pacemaker regulates the ventricular rate with no further requirement for antiarrhythmic agents. However, ablate and pace creates a lifelong dependence on the pacemaker, as AF continues and lifelong anticoagulation is required (see below). A few cases of sudden death

TABLE 8.10

Complications of catheter ablation

Pericardial effusion	1–2%
Cardiac tamponade	1%
Pulmonary vein stenosis	1%
Air embolism	≤ 1%
Aortic root puncture	< 1%
Myocardial infarction	< 1%
Systemic embolization	< 1%
Phrenic nerve paralysis	< 1%
Death	0.1%
Esophageal/left atrial fistula*	0.05%

*Very rare but often fatal because of the close anatomic relation between the lower esophagus and the pulmonary veins in some patients.

have been reported following the procedure. Ablate and pace is not the treatment of choice for young people, as they are then dependent on pacing with all the attendant long-term issues (see Chapter 11).

Left atrial appendage occlusion devices. Thrombosis in AF occurs mainly in the LAA and for some patients an occlusion device may be an appropriate alternative to warfarin. The LAA occlusion device is deployed in the mouth of the LAA and, after endothelialization, the patient can discontinue warfarin.

Surgical ablation (MAZE procedure). Patients with symptomatic AF undergoing open heart surgery for other reasons are potential candidates for AF ablation. Performed methodically, the MAZE procedure is highly successful at treating and preventing AF. Typically, surgical cuts or radiofrequency and/or cryoablation are delivered in a similar fashion to percutaneous AF ablation. Care must be taken to create complete lines of electrical block as any potential gaps increase the risk of developing atrial tachycardia/atypical atrial flutter.

Anticoagulation

Historically, patients with severe structural or valvular heart disease have been treated with warfarin (an oral vitamin K antagonist). For non-valvular AF, a large number of studies have looked at the optimal form of anticoagulation regimen and type. A meta-analysis according to the principle of intention to treat showed that adjusted-dose oral anticoagulation is highly effective for prevention of all stroke (both ischemic and hemorrhagic), with a risk reduction of 61% (95% confidence interval 47–71%) compared with placebo. Maximum protection against ischemic stroke in AF is achieved with an international normalized ratio (INR) of 2–3. An INR lower than this is not effective.

Elderly patients with AF form a special group. Dementia, recurrent falls and polypharmacy may mitigate against the use of powerful anticoagulation and each case should be judged on its own merits. Anticoagulation regimens for different patient groups are outlined in Table 8.11.

Warfarin requires regular monitoring of the INR, and drug and dietary interactions are common. If necessary, its anticoagulant effects can be quickly and effectively reversed with vitamin K (as well as plasma and/or

TABLE 8.11

Anticoagulation regimens according to patient group

Condition	Age	Regimen
Lone atrial fibrillation	< 65 years*	No anticoagulation
NVAF, $CHA_2DS_2VASc = 0$	Any age	No anticoagulation
NVAF, $CHA_2DS_2VASc \geq 1$	Any age[†]	Warfarin INR 2–3
		Dabigatran, for dose see text
		Rivaroxiban, 20 mg od
		Apixaban, 5 mg bd
Structural or valvular heart disease; previous TIA; systemic hypertension (controlled); diabetes	Any age[†]	Warfarin INR 2–3

Note: dosages for drugs are guidelines only and careful attention is required on a case-by-case basis.
*Irrespective of sex. [†]In patients over 85 years old, warfarin use should be individualized and used with caution because of a narrow benefit:risk ratio.
bd, twice daily; CHA_2DS_2Vasc, see pages 81–2; INR, international normalized ratio; NVAF, non-valvular atrial fibrillation; od, once daily; TIA, transient ischemic attack.

TABLE 8.12

Comparative pharmacology of anticoagulants

Characteristic	Warfarin	Rivaroxaban	Apixaban	Dabigatran
Target	VKORC1	Factor Xa	Factor Xa	Thrombin
Prodrug	No	No	No	Yes
Bioavailability	100%	60–80%*	60%	6%
Dosing	od	od (bd)	bd	bd (od)
Time to peak effect	4–5 days	2–4 hours	1–2 hours	1–3 hours
Half-life	40 hours	7–11 hours	12 hours	8–15 hours
Renal clearance	None	33%	25%	80%
Monitoring	Yes	No	No	No
Interactions	Multiple	3A4/P-gp	3A4/P-gp	P-gp

*Bioavailability of rivaroxaban decreases as the dose is increased because of poor drug solubility; 20 mg and 10 mg od doses have a bioavailability of 60% and 80%, respectively. 3A4, cytochrome P450 3A4 enzyme; bd, twice daily; od, once daily; P-gp, P-glycoprotein; VKORC1, C1 subunit of the vitamin K epoxide reductase enzyme. Reprinted from Weitz JI, Gross PL. *Hematology Am Soc Hematol Educ Program* 2012;2012:536–40, with permission from the American Society of Hematology.

prothrombin complex concentrates). New oral anticoagulants have been recently introduced for clinical use (Table 8.12). They have all shown non-inferiority compared with warfarin and a better safety profile, particularly with less risk of intracranial hemorrhage (Figure 8.11). However, the lack of specific antidotes for these drugs may deter both physicians and patients from using them. Efficacy, safety and costs will determine to what extent the new anticoagulants are used in clinical practice over the next few years, but the use of warfarin for non-valvular AF will decrease.

New anticoagulants include dabigatran, an oral direct thrombin inhibitor, and rivaroxiban and apixaban, factor Xa inhibitors. Newer agents such as edoxaban and betrixaban are in development.

Dabigatran is now licensed in many countries; it is not subject to dietary interactions and does not require venous monitoring. In clinical trials, a dose of 110 mg twice daily was as effective as warfarin at preventing strokes with fewer hemorrhages; at 150 mg the hemorrhage rate was

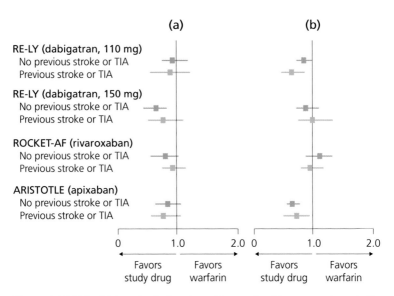

Figure 8.11 Risk of (a) stroke (ischemic and hemorrhagic) or systemic embolism and (b) major bleeding (as defined in each study), according to previous stroke or transient ischemic attack, for the new anticoagulant drugs dabigatran, rivaroxaban and apixaban versus warfarin. Reprinted from Alberts MJ et al. *Lancet Neurol* 2012;11:1066–81, with permission from Elsevier.

similar to warfarin but stroke prevention was superior. Dabigatran interacts with several drugs including verapamil and amiodarone, requiring dose adjustments. Patients with mild (50–80 mL/min creatinine clearance) or moderate (30–50 mL/min) renal impairment were included in the trials; however, dabigatran should not be used in patients with severe (< 30 mL/min) renal failure. Recommended dosages vary between countries; in general, 150 mg twice daily is suitable for patients under 75 years old with normal or mildly impaired renal function (glomerular filtration rate > 30 mL/min) and over 60 kg in weight, while 110 mg twice daily can be used in patients over 75 years old or weighing less than 60 kg (it should be noted that the 110-mg dose is not approved in the USA). Health regulatory agencies are currently working to determine whether reports of bleeding in patients taking dabigatran are more common than would be expected. Thus far there is no specific antidote to dabigatran.

Rivaroxaban and apixaban have also demonstrated efficacy in terms of stroke reduction. Rivaroxaban, 20 mg once daily, is the first oral anticoagulant in the USA that can be given once daily for AF without anticoagulation monitoring. It can be reversed with prothrombin complex. Use of rivaroxaban should be restricted in patients with severe renal impairment (creatinine clearance < 15mL/min). It has also been licensed with a boxed warning that patients should not discontinue the drug before talking to a healthcare professional, as there is an increased risk of stroke when it is discontinued. Meanwhile, a clinical trial of apixaban, 5 mg twice daily, in patients with AF who had failed or were not candidates for VKA therapy, demonstrated a reduction in the risk of stroke or systemic embolism by more than 50% compared with acetylsalicylic acid (ASA; aspirin), 81–324 mg once daily (from 3.7% per year with ASA to 1.6% per year with apixaban). Both rivaroxaban and apixaban are approved for use in patients with non-valvular AF in the USA and Europe.

Complications. Patient age and the intensity of anticoagulation are the most powerful predictors of major bleeding. The risks of anticoagulation begin to outweigh the benefits once patients reach 85 years of age (see Table 8.11). Amiodarone and propafenone potentiate, sometimes dramatically, the effects of warfarin. Such drug interactions must be considered and warfarin dosage adjusted where necessary. Use of the new anticoagulants in patients undergoing surgery requires close monitoring.

Anticoagulation for cardioversion. Although there are few randomized studies of antithrombotic therapy, it appears that the risk of thromboembolism is 1–5%. There is no solid clinical evidence that cardioversion of AF followed by prolonged maintenance of sinus rhythm effectively reduces thromboembolism. Patients with LAA thrombus are at high risk of thromboembolism after cardioversion of AF or atrial flutter. Anticoagulation should be given when AF has been present for 48 hours or more. Patients considered for cardioversion should receive anticoagulation with warfarin or dabigatran for at least 4, preferably 6, weeks beforehand. Conversion to sinus rhythm results in mechanical dysfunction of the left atrium, known as 'stunning'. This occurs after spontaneous, pharmacological or electrical conversion. Recovery of full mechanical function can take weeks and partly depends on the prior duration of the AF. The reduction in atrial function increases the risk of thromboembolism; thus, anticoagulation must be continued for a minimum of 4 weeks after cardioversion.

Key points – atrial fibrillation

- Atrial fibrillation (AF) is very common and is a major cause of morbidity and mortality.
- It is vital to determine whether AF is paroxysmal, persistent, long-standing persistent or permanent because the treatment aims are completely different for each patient group.
- Stroke risk and major bleeding risk in AF are multifactorial and can be assessed by the $CHADS_2$/CHA_2DS_2VASc and HAS-BLED scores, respectively.
- Warfarin remains the main form of anticoagulant therapy but new anticoagulants with superior or equivalent stroke reduction are emerging.
- Radiofrequency ablation (RFA) is now a feasible option for many patients with AF.
- AF ablation is still evolving as an interventional procedure, with the arrival of new mapping software and the continual evaluation of ablation methods and techniques.
- In most patients, AF is not cured by ablation. In many patients, AF is a progressive condition that may be associated with long-term recurrences of AF after apparently successful ablation procedures.

Key references

Calkins H, Kuck KH, Cappato R et al. 2012 HRS/EHRA/ECAS expert consensus statement on catheter and surgical ablation of atrial fibrillation: recommendations for patient selection, procedural techniques, patient management and follow-up, definitions, endpoints and research trial design. *Heart Rhythm* 2012;9:632–717.

Camm AJ, Kirchhof P, Lip GY et al. Guidelines for the management of atrial fibrillation (ESC 2010). *Eur Heart J* 2010;31:2369–429.

Camm AJ, Lip GY, De Caterina R et al. 2012 focused update of the ESC Guidelines for the management of atrial fibrillation: an update of the 2010 ESC Guidelines for the management of atrial fibrillation. *Eur Heart J* 2012;33:2719–47. Available at www.escardio.org/guidelines-surveys/esc-guidelines/GuidelinesDocuments/Guidelines_Focused_Update_Atrial_Fib_FT.pdf, last accessed 09 April 2013.

Camm J. 'Atrial fibrillation – an end to the epidemic?' *Circulation* 2005;112:iii.

Connolly SJ, Eikelboom J, Joyner C et al. Apixaban in patients with atrial fibrillation. *N Engl J Med* 2011;364:806–17.

Connolly SJ, Ezekowitz MD, Yusuf S et al. Dabigatran versus warfarin in patients with atrial fibrillation. *N Engl J Med* 2009;361:1139–51.

Fitzmaurice DA, Hobbs FD, Jowett S et al. Screening versus routine practice in detection of atrial fibrillation in patients aged 65 or over: cluster randomised controlled trial. *BMJ* 2007;335:.

Garcia D, Hylek E. Stroke prevention in elderly patients with atrial fibrillation. *Lancet* 2007;370:460–1.

Hohnloser SH, Crijns HJ, van Eickels M et al. Effect of dronedarone on cardiovascular events in atrial fibrillation. *N Engl J Med* 2009;360:668–78.

Hylek EM, Singer DE. Risk factors for intracranial hemorrhage in outpatients taking warfarin. *Ann Intern Med* 1994;120:897–902.

Kirchhof P, Auricchio A, Bax J et al. Outcome parameters for trials in atrial fibrillation: executive summary. Recommendations from a consensus conference organized by the German Atrial Fibrillation Competence NETwork (AFNET) and the European Heart Rhythm Association (EHRA). *Eur Heart J* 2007;28:2803–17.

Lip GY, Frison L, Halperin JL, Lane DA. Comparative validation of a novel risk score for predicting bleeding risk in anticoagulated patients with atrial fibrillation: the HAS-BLED score. *J Am Coll Cardiol* 2011;57:173–80.

Lip GY, Nieuwlaat R, Pisters R et al. Refining clinical risk stratification for predicting stroke and thromboembolism in atrial fibrillation using a novel risk factor-based approach: The Euro Heart Survey on Atrial Fibrillation. *Chest* 2010;137:263–72.

Patel MR, Mahaffey KW, Garg J et al. Rivaroxaban versus warfarin in nonvalvular atrial fibrillation. *N Engl J Med* 2011;365:883–91.

Pisters R, Lane DA, Nieuwlaat R et al. A novel user-friendly score (HAS-BLED) to assess 1-year risk of major bleeding in patients with atrial fibrillation: the Euro Heart study. *Chest* 2010; 138:1093–100.

Schnabel RB, Sullivan LM, Levy D et al. Development of a risk score for atrial fibrillation (Framingham Heart Study): a community-based cohort study. *Lancet* 2009;373:739–45.

Singer DE, Albers GW, Dalen JE et al. Antithrombotic therapy in atrial fibrillation: American College of Chest Physicians Evidence-Based Clinical Practice Guidelines (8th Edition). *Chest* 2008;133(6 Suppl):546S–92S.

Tan HW, Wang X, Shi H et al. Efficacy, safety and outcome of catheter ablation for atrial fibrillation in octogenarians. *Int J Cardiol* 2010;145:147–8.

Wilber DJ, Pappone C, Neuzil P et al. Comparison of antiarrhythmic drug therapy and radiofrequency catheter ablation in patients with paroxysmal atrial fibrillation: a randomized controlled trial. *JAMA* 2010;303: 333–40.

9 Ventricular arrhythmias

Definition

In normal conduction, the QRS complex is narrow because of near simultaneous depolarization of the ventricles, with electrical activity in the ventricles normally completing in less than 100 ms (see Figure 1.1). This rapid ventricular activation can only occur if the specialized conduction tissue within the His-Purkinje network is functioning properly. A wide QRS can occur if:

- the specialized conducting tissue is not functioning normally – bundle branch block in which depolarization of the His-Purkinje system is still from the top down but the conduction system is damaged (e.g. atrial flutter with bundle branch block will be a wide complex tachycardia)
- the specialized conducting tissue is working but is being bypassed – ventricular pre-excitation (e.g. Wolff–Parkinson–White syndrome)
- the impulses arise in the ventricle away from the His-Purkinje tissue – ventricular tachycardia (VT).

VT can be classified according to its morphology as either monomorphic (uniform) in which all the beats match each other in each lead of a surface ECG, or polymorphic (non-uniform) in which the morphology of each beat varies. There is a particular form of polymorphic VT associated with bradycardia and increased QT interval, with a cyclic progressive change in cardiac axis referred to by its French name *torsades de pointes* ('twisting of the points') (Figure 9.1).

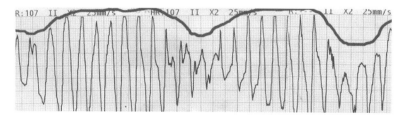

Figure 9.1 Surface ECG of *torsades de pointes*, showing the characteristic twist of the QRS complex around the isoelectric baseline.

Pathophysiology

VT may arise through different mechanisms:

- as a reflection of re-entry within an area of scar caused by infarction, ischemia or cardiomyopathy (see Figure 2.9)
- as a focal abnormality in a structurally normal heart
- because of a diffuse electrical abnormality at the cellular level (e.g. long-QT syndrome or Brugada syndrome; see Chapter 10).

In the emergency room

It is vital that a simplistic approach is taken in the emergency room:

A wide QRS complex is VT until proven otherwise

It is important a patient is not made worse when treatment is initiated following the diagnosis. Sadly, however, patients are occasionally made worse by treating a wide-QRS tachycardia as if it were arising in the atria and being conducted with bundle branch block (aberration). Agents such as intravenous verapamil can prove disastrous if the rhythm is actually VT. It is therefore generally safer to assume that all regular-QRS tachycardias are VT and to initiate treatment on that basis in the first instance. (A patient with supraventricular tachycardia [SVT] treated for VT may not get better immediately but is unlikely to get worse.)

In the occasional situation where there is strong suspicion that the rhythm is arising above the AV node, administration of intravenous adenosine can be useful in clarifying the diagnosis. If the tachycardia continues, the diagnosis is likely to be VT; if the rhythm terminates or slows with the development of AV block, an aberrantly conducted SVT is likely. Usually this diagnostic challenge is not necessary though, as knowledge of simple clinical features, such as whether the patient has had a previous myocardial infarction (MI), makes VT likely.

Emergency treatment. The choice between an electrical or drug approach is based on the clinical condition of the patient, not on the appearance of the ECG.

If the patient is hemodynamically compromised, rapid direct-current (DC) cardioversion is appropriate, although sedation or anesthesia will be needed if the patient is conscious. Once the patient is stabilized other investigations are mandatory to ascertain the best long-term treatment.

111

The arrhythmia usually identifies the presence of a significant arrhythmia substrate and continuing arrhythmia risk, and potentially sudden death. The patient should therefore be referred to an electrophysiology (EP) center for consideration of an implantable cardioverter defibrillator (ICD) or possibly ablation if appropriate (see below).

If the patient is not hemodynamically compromised, administration of an agent such as lidocaine (lignocaine) or amiodarone is appropriate. Lidocaine, up to 1.5 mg/kg administered over 10 minutes, has a modest efficacy (approximately 30% success) and is the least negatively inotropic of the class 1 antiarrhythmic agents. Amiodarone has multiple antiarrhythmic actions and is the most potent agent for VT currently available. The oral form has minimal negative inotropic action but the diluent in some intravenous forms of the drug may cause significant hypotension. It should be administered as a slow bolus of 300 mg over 30 minutes via a central vein (or large antecubital vein). If continuing antiarrhythmic action is required, an infusion of 900–1500 mg over 24 hours may be necessary.

If these agents fail, it is better to resort early to DC cardioversion rather than to reach for further antiarrhythmic drugs that may worsen cardiac performance in the long term, either because of a deleterious effect on myocardial contractility (negative inotropism) or by provoking new arrhythmias (proarrhythmic action) – see Chapter 5.

General treatment principles

Although ventricular arrhythmias may occur in the context of an acute transient event such as during an acute MI, generally whenever VT occurs two problems dominate the overall management of the patient: the arrhythmia may recur and it may degenerate to ventricular fibrillation (VF) and sudden death.

The therapeutic options depend on the likelihood of recurrence and on the mechanism involved, which influences the risk of sudden death. The key questions to consider in managing a patient with VT are:
- does the patient have a continuing propensity for the arrhythmia?
- does this arrhythmia reflect structural heart disease?

VT in the structurally normal heart

Diagnosis. Patients occasionally complain of exercise-induced palpitations, with symptoms typically emerging just after vigorous exercise. The typical form is due to early depolarizations provoked by catecholamines leading to repetitive firing from an area within the outflow tract. It is crucial to recognize the different variants from the 12-lead ECG so that detailed mapping can be performed in the correct area.

Exercise-induced right ventricular outflow tract (RVOT) tachycardia must also be distinguished from arrhythmogenic right ventricular cardiomyopathy, which is a scar-related, often progressive, condition that may ultimately require an ICD. Distinguishing features are shown in Figure 9.2.

Rarely, patients may present with idiopathic left VT or fascicular VT with a characteristic ECG pattern that arises in, or very close, to the specialized conducting tissue in the left ventricle (often the QRS complexes during the arrhythmia are not too wide). The commonest site is the posterior fascicle, which presents with right-bundle left-axis VT (Figure 9.3). The VT is most often seen in men, is occasionally exercise related and may show sensitivity to calcium-channel blockers.

Management. If the patient has a structurally normal heart and the arrhythmia is a 'normal heart VT' they can be treated symptomatically, using medication such as beta-blockers or curative catheter ablation

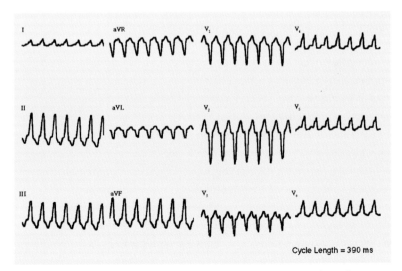

Cycle Length = 390 ms

Figure 9.2 12-lead ECG of typical right ventricular outflow tract (RVOT) tachycardia. Note the positive complexes in II, III and aVF, and the R wave transition between V3 and V4.

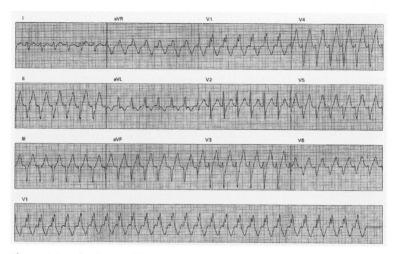

Figure 9.3 12-lead ECG of fascicular ventricular tachycardia. Typical right-bundle, left-axis morphology with a relatively narrow QRS.

(which has become the treatment of choice for this focal arrhythmia). Providing the patient is not syncopal, sudden death is rare.

Antiarrhythmic drugs are gradually falling out of favor because of their generic side effects (negative inotropism and proarrhythmia; see Chapter 5) and because non-drug options are superior.

Mapping and ablation. The 'normal heart VTs' are usually autonomically dependent and may be difficult to induce during EP study; heavy sedation or general anesthesia may render them completely non-inducible. In some cases isoprenaline (isoproterenol) infusion is required to induce the arrhythmia. Even if it is inducible, the VT may not be sustained and so prolonged mapping of the arrhythmia may not be possible. If the VT can be sustained, then conventional activation mapping is performed, using the earliest endocardial signal as the point of ablation.

If VT cannot be reliably sustained then an alternative strategy is pace-mapping. The pattern of ventricular myocardial depolarization occurs in a particular way as it spreads from the focal source to the rest of the myocardium, producing a characteristic 12-lead ECG pattern. If a catheter is placed at this same site and pacing is performed, the 12-lead ECG morphology will look identical only if it is in the same place as the VT source. During ablation at the correct site there is often an accelerated burst of VT (automaticity), which is extinguished during continued ablation. The main advantage of this technique is that it only requires a single abnormal beat to be recorded and hence is useful even if the rhythm is difficult to induce or sustain.

Rarely, VT may arise in association with the fascicles of the His-Purkinje system, particularly the left posterior fascicle. The VT has a characteristic 12-lead morphology with a relatively narrow right-bundle left-axis appearance (see Figure 9.3). The VT is calcium dependent and hence verapamil sensitive, and is best treated by catheter ablation.

VT with structural heart disease. Patients with evidence of myocardial scarring or a diffuse electrical abnormality are at significant risk of further episodes and sudden death. Occasionally, patients with these conditions present with VT storms with frequent episodes of polymorphic VT or VF that are difficult to manage and may require multiple DC shocks.

Management. Beta-blockers and amiodarone are usually started, and are the mainstay of treatment, but occasionally patients continue to have recurrent episodes despite treatment. The degree of LV dysfunction is an important risk stratifier, and all cases should be mandatorily referred for assessment for an ICD. The ICD is extremely effective in a secondary prevention role and is the cornerstone of treatment. ICDs are also highly effective as a primary preventive strategy (see Chapter 11).

Ablation. Unlike VTs in the normal heart, where catheter ablation is often curative, the procedure has been traditionally viewed as palliative in patients with structural heart disease, particularly in conditions such as arrhythmogenic right ventricular cardiomyopathy where there may be significant disease progression with time. However, catheter ablation can be effective at reducing or eliminating ICD shocks in patients with scar-related VT. The ablation strategy is very different from SVT ablation (Table 9.1).

TABLE 9.1

Differences between catheter ablation in scar-related ventricular tachycardia (VT) and supraventricular tachycardia (SVT)

SVT ablation	Scar-related VT ablation
Point ablation	Linear or area ablation
Small residual endocardial scar ($\leq$ 4 mm)	Deep transmural lesions
> 95% success	60–70% success
Isolated electrical abnormality	Arrhythmia must be considered with the associated heart disease (e.g. heart failure, ischemia)
Clear endpoint	Endpoint difficult
Complex mapping systems helpful	Complex mapping systems essential
Low-risk procedure	Increased risks (e.g. stroke)
Often curative	Palliative – may recur over time

Key points – ventricular tachycardia

- A wide regular QRS complex indicates ventricular tachycardia (VT) until proven otherwise.
- All patients with a wide complex tachycardia need emergency referral and admission
- VT may occur in a structurally normal heart and tends to show characteristic ECG and clinical features.
- Catheter ablation is curative for normal-heart VT but palliative for scar-related VT.
- Wide-QRS tachycardia always requires further investigation and referral to an arrhythmia specialist.

An arrhythmia forms a significant component of a number of unusual syndromes. These syndromes have some features in common: they are rare, many have eponymous titles, and they often have a genetic component, either recognized or surmised, and are usually familial.

Ion channelopathies

Normal mechanisms that control the movement of ions through channels (sodium, potassium and calcium) are responsible for effective myocyte function. Genetic mutations produce abnormalities in these channels, which affect the behavior of ions and thus produce an electrical disturbance in the myocytes. In some cases this leads to an arrhythmia that can cause sudden death in an apparently healthy individual with a structurally normal heart. These arrhythmias are very often episodic. Patients can have long periods between arrhythmic events. As a group these syndromes are referred to as channelopathies, and include the long- and short-QT syndromes and Brugada syndrome.

Long-QT syndromes. The normal QT interval (measured from the onset of the Q wave to the end of the T wave) in the 12-lead ECG is 380–460 ms, and reflects both depolarization and repolarization (see Chapter 1). A long QT interval (or, rarely, a pathologically short QT interval) predisposes an individual to ventricular arrhythmias, usually a polymorphic (non-uniform) ventricular tachycardia (VT) known as *torsades de pointes*. The QT interval shortens as the heart rate increases and lengthens with bradycardias. Thus, to allow comparison of the QT intervals at different heart rates, the QT interval is rate-corrected (QTc) by dividing the QT by the square root of the R-R interval. In the long-QT syndrome (LQTS), both potassium and sodium channels are affected, resulting in prolonged repolarization.

   Congenital long-QT syndrome is an inherited disorder characterized by prolonged ventricular repolarization on the ECG and a propensity to ventricular arrhythmias. Syncope and sudden death may result from *torsades de pointes*. This VT with an undulating axis may degenerate into

117

ventricular fibrillation (VF), leading to death. *Torsades de pointes* is typically initiated by sudden increases in sympathetic tone such as that triggered by fright, stress or physical exertion.

The prevalence of LQTS is approximately 1 in 4000 in the general population, with the onset of symptoms typically occurring within the first two decades of life. Presentation may vary from merely prolongation of the QT interval noted on the 12-lead ECG in an asymptomatic individual to recurrent syncope or resuscitated sudden death. Many patients are initially labeled as having epilepsy.

Several forms of congenital LQTS have been described; three forms have been well characterized (LQT1, LQT2 , LQT3). These forms have distinct clinical outcomes, ECG appearances (Figure 10.1) and triggers. Most commonly, sudden death in LQT1 is seen after physical exertion (e.g. in athletes), in LQT2 sudden death or syncope is usually seen during emotional stress and in LQT3 sudden death can occur during sleep.

Treatment modalities include:

- beta-blockade
- pacing
- implantable cardioverter defibrillator (ICD)
- cardiac sympathectomy
- mexiletine (in LQT3).

Beta-blockade abolishes symptoms in 80% of cases, although it is less effective in LQT3. In many cases beta-blockade produces significant

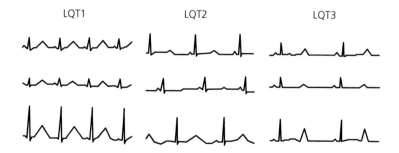

Figure 10.1 ECGs showing three forms of long-QT syndrome: LQT1 in which the T wave is long in duration; LQT2 in which the T wave is small and notched; and LQT3 in which the T wave has a long onset. Although the arrhythmia risk is higher in LQT1 and LQT2 the risk of death is higher in LQT3.

bradycardia (which itself increases the QT interval); these cases benefit from additional pacing, usually within the atria only. Pacing at a relatively high rate (80–100 bpm) keeps the QT short. In rare cases an ICD is required, although this is often a last resort because patients are mostly children. Cardiac sympathectomy was used in early cases but has been largely superseded by more effective treatments.

Acquired long-QT syndrome is most commonly either drug induced or due to a profound biochemical abnormality, usually hypocalcemia or hypomagnesemia. Drugs that prolong the QT interval are shown in Table 10.1. It should be remembered that by their very action some antiarrhythmic drugs prolong the QT interval. This does not mean the drug should be stopped. As a rule, if the QTc (see page 117) is greater than 500 ms then it is advisable to withdraw treatment because of the unpredictable occurrence of *torsades de pointes*. Antiarrhythmic agents

TABLE 10.1

Drugs that prolong the QT interval

Cardiac drugs
- Quinidine
- Procainamide
- Disopyramide
- Amiodarone
- Sotalol
- Bretylium

Psychotropic agents
- Thioridazine
- Chlorpromazine
- Haloperidol
- Tricyclic antidepressants
- Lithium
- Sertindole
- Zotepine

Antimalarials/antibiotics
- Erythromycin
- Pentamidine
- Halofantrine
- Amantadine
- Quinine
- Chloroquine

Serotonin antagonists
- Ketanserin

Others
- Probucol
- Vasopressin
- Terfanidine
- Astemizole
- Tacrolimus

capable of prolonging the QT interval should not be used together. Large biochemical variations, particularly hypo- or hyperkalemia or hypocalcemia, should be avoided. Potassium levels should be checked regularly in patients on diuretic therapy and in those with intercurrent illness such as severe diarrhea.

Over the years, many drugs have been withdrawn from general use because of complications associated with QT prolongation and increased risk of sudden death (e.g. cisapride, terodiline). A comprehensive list of drugs that prolong the QT interval and/or induce *torsades de pointes* can be found at www.azcert.org/medical-pros/drug-lists/CLQTS.cfm.

Brugada syndrome was first described by the Brugada brothers in 1992. It is a rare syndrome characterized by sudden death due to idiopathic VF in an otherwise apparently structurally normal heart. More than 80 mutations in the sodium-channel gene have been identified in patients with Brugada syndrome. The arrhythmias are believed to be mainly due to differences in repolarization in regions of the epicardium at the right ventricular outflow tract (RVOT), allowing re-entry to occur. The diagnostic ECG abnormality is shown in Figure 10.2. Brugada syndrome is known as Lai Tai in Thailand; in other parts of Asia (e.g. Philippines, Japan), the condition is one of the most common causes of natural death in men under 50 years of age. An ICD is the treatment of choice in patients with syncope, resuscitated sudden death or inducible ventricular arrhythmias. Electrophysiological (EP) testing may be useful in asymptomatic cases (e.g. patients in whom Brugada syndrome is found incidentally) to assess the risk of sudden death.

Confusingly, the ECG changes (post-prandial, fever) are intermittent in some patients and a high index of suspicion is required to make the diagnosis. Patients with documented VF with an otherwise normal heart should undergo a provocation test using intravenous administration of a sodium-channel blocker such as ajmaline (a short-acting class 1 agent) or flecainide during 12-lead ECG recording. This brings out or exaggerates the ECG changes, confirming the diagnosis.

Lists of drugs that should be avoided by patients with Brugada syndrome can be found at www.brugadadrugs.org.

Patients presenting with resuscitated sudden death are at highest risk of recurrence. Among asymptomatic patients, those with intermittent

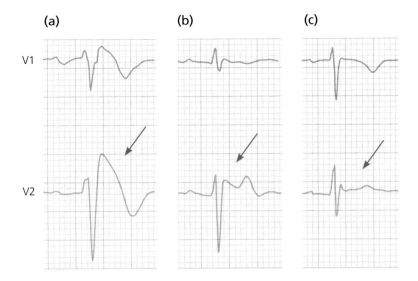

Figure 10.2 Characteristic appearance of the ECG in types 1, 2 and 3 Brugada syndrome. (a) Type 1 is a coved-type ST-segment elevation (J wave) of ≥ 2 mm or 0.2 mV at its peak, followed by a negative T wave with little or no isoelectric separation, and is pathognomonic of Brugada syndrome. (b) Type 2 is a saddle-back ST-segment elevation of ≥ 2 mm (a gradually descending ST-segment elevation followed by a positive T wave). (c) Type 3 is a right precordial ST-segment elevation (saddle-back type, coved type, or both).

Brugada ECGs or with ECG appearances with class 1 antiarrhythmic agents are at neglible risk for arrhythmic events. The role of EP testing has been debated; it is used predominantly to assess the risk of sudden death.

Arrhythmogenic right ventricular cardiomyopathy

Arrhythmogenic right ventricular cardiomyopathy (ARVC) is a rare but important cause of VT and sudden death, particularly in young men; in particular, it causes tachycardia on vigorous exercise. ARVC is due to genetic abnormalities in the desmosome regions of myocytes (the desmosomes link cardiac cells and confer strength). The hypothesis is that in these regions mechanical stress causes cell death (and the process may be accelerated by vigorous endurance exercise). Cell death is followed by fibrofatty replacement of myocardial tissue in three regions of the right ventricle where the wall stresses are greatest. This produces areas of slow conduction, as islands of surviving myocardium are separated by scar tissue, which in turn favors re-entry and the development of VT.

Hypertrophic cardiomyopathy

Hypertrophic cardiomyopathy (HCM) is a spectrum of disorders that affects myocardial structure, including asymmetric septal hypertrophy and idiopathic subaortic stenosis. Abnormal myocardial architecture and fiber disarray contribute to increased risk of VF in patients with HCM. Five factors have been associated with an increased risk of sudden death, and such patients should be considered for an ICD:

- recurrent syncope
- non-sustained VT on ambulatory ECG monitoring
- little (< 10 mmHg) or no blood pressure response with exercise
- interventricular septal thickness > 3 cm
- family history of sudden death.

Catecholaminergic polymorphic ventricular tachycardia

Catecholaminergic polymorphic ventricular tachycardia (CPVT) is a rare genetic abnormality, first described in children, which causes syncope and sudden death due to bidirectional or polymorphic VT following exercise or stress. It is caused by abnormalities in intramyocardial calcium handling, usually due to mutations in the genes that code for either the ryanodine receptor or calsequestrin. Beta receptor blockade either by a maximal dose of beta-blockers or sympathetic denervation is crucial but may not be fully protective, and additional agents such as flecainide may be useful.

Genetics and sudden death

Although there is evidence of coronary disease in 80% of cases of sudden death and some form of cardiomyopathy in 5%, no clear structural defect is found in up to a third of postmortems in sudden death cases.

In the event of an unexplained sudden cardiac death, particularly at a young age, the possibility of a genetic cause should be considered and investigated. Unfortunately, only a small percentage of carriers of an abnormal gene (e.g. Brugada syndrome) will have an abnormal ECG, and current clinical tests (e.g. MRI) are not sufficiently reliable to be clinically useful. However, genetic screening can be very helpful in conditions where the genetic basis is clear and testing is robust. Screening and counseling of family members should be carried out at specialized centers, with clear communication and referral systems in place between diagnostic testers, community healthcare providers, coroner services and affected families.

Key points – rare and inherited arrhythmias

- An arrhythmic cause should be considered in younger patients presenting with 'epilepsy' – a resting ECG is mandatory.
- ECG changes may be intermittent; a normal baseline ECG may not exclude these conditions.
- Several forms of congenital long-QT syndrome have been described, the most well-characterized of which – LQT1, LQT2 and LQT3 – each have distinct clinical outcomes, ECG appearances and triggers.
- Brugada syndrome is characterized by sudden death due to idiopathic VF; ECG changes may be intermittent, but an abnormality resembling incomplete or complete right bundle branch block pattern with persistent ST elevation in the precordial chest leads (V1–V3) is diagnostic.
- Most cases of long-QT syndrome are drug related.
- Patients with known hypertrophic cardiomyopathy require cardiologic assessment.
- In many cases screening of family members is mandatory and, if available, referral to a specialized genetics clinic should be made.

Key reference

Marcus FI, McKenna WJ, Sherrill D et al. Diagnosis of arrhythmogenic right ventricular cardiomyopathy/dysplasia: proposed modification of the task force criteria. *Circulation* 2010;121:1533–41.

The superiority of device therapy over long-term drug therapy is now well established. Cardiac devices are the mainstay of treatment for patients with bradycardias, ventricular tachyarrhythmias and some types of heart failure.

Pacemakers

Approximately 25 000 pacemakers are implanted in the UK every year. Worldwide the rate of pacemaker implants varies widely: 752 per million in the USA, 550 in Canada, 590 in Australia and 447 in the UK.

Indications. Pacemakers are the treatment of choice for pathological bradycardias and heart blocks, as described below.

Bradyarrhythmia is the main reason for pacemaker implantation. It is defined as a heart beat that is too slow, usually less than 60 bpm, and causes symptoms. However, for some people (e.g. athletes) a low heart rate, particularly at rest, may be normal. Some patients with bradyarrhythmia are asymptomatic but common symptoms include fatigue, dizziness, syncope and breathlessness (see Chapter 3). The two most common types of bradyarrhythmia are sick sinus syndrome and atrioventricular (AV) block.

Sick sinus syndrome, also known as sinus node disease, affects the generation of the action potential by the sinus node. It is characterized by severe sinus bradycardia, sinus pauses or arrest (often greater than 3 seconds), atrial tachyarrhythmias (paroxysms of atrial fibrillation [AF] and/or flutter) with alternating periods of atrial bradyarrhythmias and sometimes inappropriate responses of heart rate during exercise or stress (Figure 11.1). Although it can occur at any age, incidence increases exponentially with age. The mean age of patients with the syndrome is 68 years, with similar numbers of men and women being affected. The syndrome occurs in 1 of every 600 cardiac patients older than 65 years and accounts for approximately half of all pacemaker implants. It is also common for patients to receive multiple antiarrhythmic drug therapies,

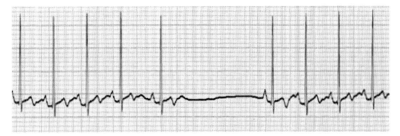

Figure 11.1 Rhythm strip showing a series of normal sinus beats followed by a failure of the sinus node (sinus pause) with resumption of normal sinus rhythm thereafter. Pauses can be very long (occasionally 20–30 seconds) causing presyncope and syncope in some patients.

which often exacerbate any tendency to bradycardia. Sinus pauses of more than 5 seconds in patients with presyncope or syncope usually require pacing.

Atrioventricular block can be categorized as first-, second- or third-degree (complete) heart block. Heart block in one of these forms accounts for 40–60% of patients who have pacemakers implanted.

First-degree block is defined as a PR interval of greater than 200 ms (five small squares on a surface ECG; Figure 11.2a). Rarely, symptomatic patients may require pacing. There are two types of second-degree block.

- In Mobitz type I block (also known as the Wenckebach phenomenon) there is a gradual progressive lengthening of the PR interval in sinus rhythm, culminating in a dropped beat (Figure 11.2b). This type of second-degree block often does not require pacing. The condition is usually transient, related to infarction or ischemia, or occasionally is drug induced.
- In Mobitz type II block there is no lengthening of the PR interval in sinus rhythm but a sudden dropped beat (i.e. no conducted QRS complex; Figure 11.2c). Pacing is mandatory in these patients because of the unpredictable risk of sudden ventricular standstill.

Complete block is characterized by a slow regular ventricular response of 30–40 bpm and the sinus beats are not conducted to the ventricles (Figure 11.2d). There is no mathematical relationship between the rate of the P waves and the rate of the QRS complexes. Complete heart block may be congenital or acquired. Acquired heart block always requires pacing. For congenital heart block the time to start pacing should be

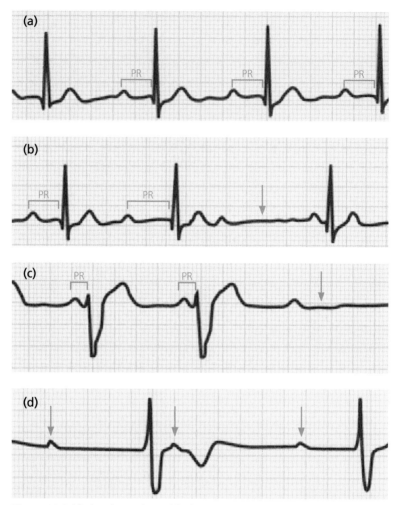

Figure 11.2 (a) First-degree heart block, with a PR interval of 200 ms.
(b) Second-degree heart block (Mobitz type I), in which the PR interval gradually
lengthens until the P wave is not conducted. The QRS is narrow. (c) Second-
degree heart block (Mobitz type II), in which the PR interval stays constant
before the dropping of a ventricular beat. The QRS is wide. (d) Complete heart
block, in which there is no association between the P waves and the QRS
compexes. The arrows show P waves that are not conducted to the ventricles.

decided on an individual basis before 40 years of age. Symptomatology is
not the major criterion for pacing: average heart rate, pauses in the

intrinsic rate, exercise tolerance, presence of maternal antibodies mediated block, and heart structure are all important. Prospective studies suggest early pacing offers a survival advantage.

Trifascicular block describes a block in all three fascicles of the His-Purkinje system. It is defined as either left bundle branch block together with first-degree block, or a combination of left anterior or posterior hemiblock, complete right bundle branch block and first-degree block (Figure 11.3). In left anterior hemiblock the QRS axis is markedly leftward; in left posterior it is markedly rightward. Prophylactic pacing is recommended. These patients usually have heart disease, other comorbidities and the conduction disease may progress to heart block.

Carotid sinus hypersensitivity (CSH) is a recognized cause of syncope and falls. CSH increases in prevalence with age and is rare in patients younger than 50 years old. It is characterized by prolonged heart-rate slowing (often with pauses in excess of 3.5 seconds – known as the cardioinhibitory type) or a profound drop in systolic blood pressure (hypotensive type) in response to carotid sinus massage (CSM). Often both are present. Where slowing of the heart rate is the predominant abnormality, cardiac pacing often reduces symptoms significantly. Varied

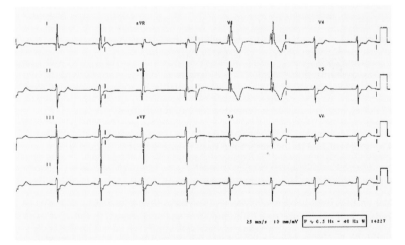

Figure 11.3 A 12-lead ECG showing trifascicular block: complete right bundle branch block (RBBB; a bifid QRS complex in V1 and V2 known as an rSr pattern), marked left axis deviation (a positive R wave in leads I and aVL) and first-degree heart block (PR interval > 200 ms).

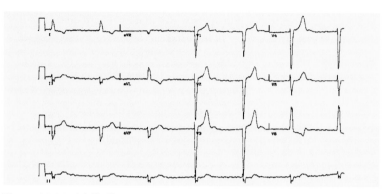

Figure 11.4 Atrial fibrillation with complete heart block. There are no visible P waves. The QRS rate is slow and regular.

responses have been due to differences in methods of recruitment of participants, settings, comorbidities, duration of CSM and definitions of abnormal responses.

Atrial fibrillation. Some patients with AF have an intermittently slow heart rate that produces symptoms of presyncope or syncope (Figure 11.4). Patients with Holter-recorded RR intervals greater than 5 seconds, even if asymptomatic, require a pacemaker. If there are pauses of more than 3 seconds with symptoms of presyncope or syncope, a pacemaker may be necessary. Frequently, drug treatment is given to slow the ventricular rate during AF and this will often exacerbate any bradycardia. In many patients such drug treatment cannot be withdrawn. Thus, a combination of antiarrhythmia medication (to slow fast heart rates during AF) and a pacemaker are not uncommon.

Heart failure. Traditionally, pacemakers were implanted exclusively for bradycardias. However, in the past 15 years heart failure without bradycardia has become a new indication. In some cases of heart failure the systolic contraction of the ventricles is not synchronous; parts of the left and right ventricles contract in an uncoordinated fashion, resulting in reduced cardiac output and functional mitral regurgitation. Often the QRS complex is broad, usually with a left bundle branch block morphology. Even with optimal pharmacological treatment with tolerated doses of beta-blockers, ACE inhibitors, diuretics and spironolactone, with or without digoxin, some patients remain symptomatic with shortness of breath and tiredness. Cardiac resynchronization therapy (CRT), also referred to as biventricular pacing (BiV-P), should be considered in patients with the following inclusion criteria:

- severe shortness of breath (NYHA grade III and ambulatory grade IV breathlessness) despite optimal medical treatment
- broad QRS complexes > 120 ms (usually sinus rhythm but also AF)
- QRS width 120–150 ms with echocardiographic evidence of cardiac dysynchrony, or QRS width > 150 ms.

A standard lead is positioned in the right ventricle, usually at the apex, and in the right atrium (during sinus rhythm). A third lead is positioned within the coronary venous system, if possible in the posterolateral vein underneath the left ventricle; a venous angiogram defines the anatomy (Figure 11.5). The right and left ventricles can then be stimulated simultaneously, resynchronizing ventricular contraction.

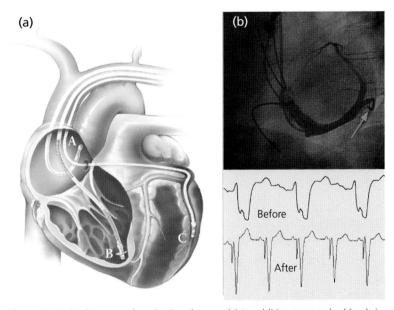

Figure 11.5 Cardiac resynchronization therapy. (a) In addition to standard leads in the right atrium (A) and at the apex of the right ventricle (B), a third lead is placed within the coronary sinus to access a posterolateral vein (C). (b) An occlusive venogram taken during implantation defines venous anatomy for placement of lead C. The posterolateral vein is usually selected (arrow). Leads B and C simultaneously pace both ventricles to resynchronize contraction of the ventricles. This usually produces a narrowing of the QRS complexes on the surface ECG.

A number of randomized international studies have shown an improvement in morbidity and quality of life, and a significant reduction in mortality. However, for reasons that are not fully understood, only approximately 75% of patients respond positively. Patients with non-ischemic cardiomyopathies usually do better. There is no convincing test that predicts who will benefit.

Implantation. The pacemaker is inserted under local anesthesia (approximately 40 mL lidocaine [lignocaine] infiltrated into the anterior chest wall and under the left or right clavicle), in a sterile operating environment, usually in a standard catheter laboratory. The patient is often given a premedication and antibiotics to reduce the possibility of infection. By convention the device is usually inserted in the left prepectoral position under the clavicle (Figure 11.6) but it can be inserted on the right side. For a standard pacemaker, the procedure usually takes 30–60 minutes; for CRT it can take up to 3–4 hours.

The pacing leads are positioned in the heart using radiographic imaging. The patient is mobilized within a few hours and allowed home the following day. Some centers perform implantation as a day-case procedure. A chest radiograph is required to document satisfactory lead position and the absence of pneumothorax. An ECG is performed to document proper capture and morphology of the QRS complex.

(a)   (b)

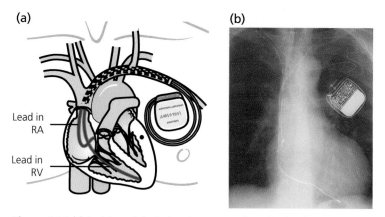

Lead in
RA

Lead in
RV

Figure 11.6 (a) Position of dual-chamber pacemaker after implantation.
(b) Radiograph of the pacemaker and atrial and ventricular leads. RA, right
atrium; RV, right ventricle.

Complications. There is often a degree of bruising around the wound and some discomfort, all usually short lived. Patients are encouraged to keep the left shoulder mobile to a degree. Fear of activity can lead to frozen shoulder.

Short-term problems. Use of the subclavian vein is associated with a 1–2% risk of pneumothorax. Hemothorax is rare, as is death. Cardiac perforation, by the pacing leads, has been described but very rarely leads to tamponade. Lead displacement following implantation can occur but is uncommon with modern leads; it is more common with atrial than ventricular leads and is often operator dependent. Acute infection is very rare as many centers now give antibiotics before the procedure.

Long-term problems. Late infection is a rare but serious complication. Infection at the pacemaker site mandates removal of the system including the generator and leads. If the patient is dependent on the pacemaker (i.e. has no underlying heart rhythm) then a temporary pacing lead is inserted and a permanent system is reimplanted when the infection has cleared. If the patient is not dependent on the pacemaker then a permanent system is reimplanted when the infection has cleared with no need for interim intervention. Pacemaker erosion is also a rare complication now that the generators are so small. Erosion is nearly always associated with infection and also requires removal of the whole system.

A broken lead needs to be either replaced or possibly removed. However, removal can be difficult if the lead has been implanted for more than a year (see lead extraction, page 142).

Product recalls. Occasionally, leads or devices have a higher than expected failure rate, in which case the manufacturer issues a product recall (see pages 142–3). In such instances, physicians are advised to monitor those patients who have had these potentially faulty products implanted more closely (e.g. follow-up every 3 months rather than once a year). Removal is not usually recommended unless it is mandated (e.g. the possibility of a sudden device failure in a patient who is dependent on pacing) or if the patient experiences device/lead-related problems.

Pacemaker function

Leads. Pacemaker leads consist of an inner metallic core through which electrical energy is delivered to the tip and thereby to the heart. This core is insulated from body fluids by an inert external synthetic coat made of either polyurethane or silicone. The tip has 'tines' that fix or 'lock' into the

131

trabeculations within the right ventricle and/or atrium, or have a mechanical method of screwing the tip into the myocardium (Figure 11.7). The lead causes a local tissue reaction and the tip eventually becomes fibrosed. The aim is to prevent displacement of the tip as a result of cardiac motion or with time.

The tip of the lead can be either unipolar or bipolar. Modern systems tend to use bipolar leads, which allow more specific sensing of the endocardial signal. Unipolar leads are more likely to pick up extraneous interference and are rarely used nowadays.

The lead body is incredibly resilient, flexing and twisting to accommodate daily cardiac contractions. Lead failure is rare (< 0.05% fracture per year) and lifespan is often 10–15 years. Fractures can occur within either the inner conducting core or the outer insulation and very rarely lead to sudden loss of pacing function. Contiguity is usually maintained even when a lead fractures internally. Lead embolization has never been reported, and internal lead erosion (i.e. through a large vein in the chest or through the heart) is very rare. Lead integrity can be assessed non-invasively via the pacemaker generator, previously on an annual basis, but newer devices are able to check lead function daily and even attempt automatic reprogramming to maintain safety. A broken lead requires replacement or, rarely, removal (see below). The pacing generator is not easily damaged, except perhaps by major trauma.

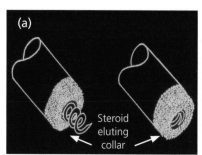
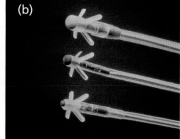

Figure 11.7 Permanent pacing lead tips. (a) Active fixation: the lead is anchored to the myocardium using a small screw. The electrically active collar (shown) is then opposed to the myocardium. The collar leaches steroids locally to prevent excessive fibrosis at the lead tip/myocardial interface. (b) Passive fixation: the tines lock themselves into the trabeculations within the walls of the right ventricle to maintain stability.

Single- and dual-chamber devices. Early pacemakers used a lead positioned in the apex of the right ventricle only, which was easy to access via the great cardiac veins in the neck and shoulders (subclavian venous system). More modern systems also pace the right atrium in order to mimic the heart's own intrinsic rhythm and maintain AV synchrony. The risk of thrombotic embolization from a lead in the right ventricle is very low compared with pacing within the left ventricle and enables reliable pacing of the heart whatever the intrinsic cardiac conduction. The right atrium can also be paced safely long term. In the presence of completely normal AV nodal function, atrial-based pacing is the mode of choice.

Coding of pacemakers is shown in Table 11.1. More complex pacemakers have the ability to sense and/or stimulate both the atria and ventricles.

TABLE 11.1

Categorization of pacemakers*

I	II	III	IV	V
Category				
Chamber(s) paced	Chamber(s) sensed	Response to sensing	Rate modulation	Multisite pacing
Letters used				
O-None	O-None	O-None	O-None	O-None
A-Atrium	A-Atrium	T-Triggered	R-Rate modulation	A-Atrium
V-Ventricle		V-Ventricle	I-Inhibited	V-Ventricle
D-Dual (A+V)	D-Dual (A+V)	D-Dual (T+1)		D-Dual (A+V)

- Position I indicates the chamber or chambers paced
- Position II indicates the chamber that senses the intrinsic signal
- Position III indicates the response to sensing
- Position IV indicates the programmable parameters of the device
- Position V indicates whether the device has any anti-tachycardia features

*According to the Heart Rhythm Society of America and Heart Rhythm UK.

Demand pacing. Very early pacemakers were life-saving devices but had two major limitations: they did not sense the underlying heart rhythm and delivered pacing impulses constantly, whether required or not (fixed-rate or asynchronous).

Modern pacemakers deliver demand pacing, the ability to sense spontaneous cardiac depolarization and to inhibit pacemaker output; they therefore work only when required (Figure 11.8), thereby extending battery life.

Cardiac sensors. Initially, demand pacemakers were only able to pace the ventricles at a constant rate (e.g. 70 pulses/minute) irrespective of the metabolic demands of the patient. Although they were life-saving, these early systems created increased morbidity. Frequent complaints were shortness of breath or exercise-induced tiredness. There are now many sensors capable of detecting changes in the physical demand of the patient. Two or three types are used as standard. Cardiac sensors detect either body movement vibration, cardiac output, respiration rate or the QT interval and allow the pacemaker's response to be tailored to the demands of the individual patient.

Programmability. In modern pacemakers, the pacing rate can be altered and the power output adjusted. In more complex systems, both the atrial and ventricular channels can be programmed independently. The endocardial signal (internal ECG) can be recorded, and with some pacemakers the patient can externally trigger the pacemaker to store these signals when they are symptomatic, acting like a cardiomemo device.

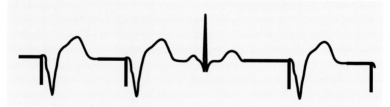

Figure 11.8 Ventricular demand pacing: the first two complexes are paced beats; the third is an intrinsic cardiac beat that has inhibited the pacemaker – there is no pacing spike. Following the intrinsic beat there is no further intrinsic beat and the pacemaker then paces to maintain the cardiac output.

Pacemakers are programmed non-invasively by placing a telemetry wand over the pacemaker and connecting this to a sophisticated computer. Radiofrequency signals are used to alter the settings, a painless process that often takes 5–10 minutes to perform.

Battery life. Programming is a balance between getting the best out of the system and device longevity. On average, modern lithium-iodide batteries last 5–10 years, depending on how often the pacemaker paces and how many complex parameters are switched on. Battery depletion is gradual, and devices very rarely fail suddenly. Battery life is monitored by the pacemaker, which alerts the programmer to battery depletion. Battery replacement is a day-case procedure.

Optimal pacing mode. A number of international large-scale randomized trials have compared different pacing modalities. In the main, atrial-based pacing is preferred if AV nodal function is intact. However, in patients with complete heart block no difference in mortality has been found between single-chamber (VVI) and dual-chamber (DDD) pacing, although the incidence of AF is lower with atrial-based pacing. For complete heart block, a rate-responsive ventricular demand pacemaker (VVIR) is as effective as DDD pacing in the elderly, but DDD pacing is still preferred in younger patients and patients with good exercise capacity. Modern pacemakers use an algorithm that minimizes the amount of ventricular pacing, thereby reducing the possibility of future heart failure (see below).

Optimal lead position. Although the right ventricular apex (RVA) has been the position of choice since the inception of pacing, recent evidence suggests that long-term pacing at the RVA can cause deterioration in LV function resulting in heart failure. There is now much interest in alternate sites for pacing, and new technology is allowing leads to be placed anywhere in the right ventricle. Currently it is not known which is the best site.

External interference. All pacemakers sense the underlying cardiac signal via sensing circuits capable of filtering, to a degree, electrical signals. Any sensing circuit will be overwhelmed if the external noise is sufficient. However, all modern systems are well shielded and considerable interference is required to alter or damage a pacemaker. Exposure to

135

high-level electromagnetic fields is unlikely during normal daily living, although any machine capable of generating a high-density current, such as an arc-welding unit, may be capable of disturbing a pacemaker. Security systems in airports and department stores are safe. In the event that a pacemaker is overwhelmed by external interference the sensing circuits are temporarily switched off and the device paces continuously until the interference is resolved. Rarely, the device will sense extrinsic noise that it interprets as an underlying QRS complex. Under these circumstances the pacemaker will inhibit its output and fail to pace, which may result in symptoms of dizziness or syncope.

Effect on quality of life

Driving. Regulations for returning to driving after pacemaker implantation vary between countries (and even between States in the USA) but, in general, patients who have had blackouts and have the cause identified and treated by a pacemaker are able to drive 1–2 weeks after the procedure. It is advisable to avoid driving for a week anyway. Any irritation at the site of implantation in the initial weeks after surgery is not an excuse not to wear a seatbelt; in such cases, padding should be used. Pacemaker implantation precludes the flying of commercial aircraft. Non-commercial pilots and drivers of heavy goods vehicles or passenger service vehicles must have their licenses assessed by the relevant authorities.

Pregnancy. Pacemakers are rarely used in women of child-bearing age. There is no contraindication to pregnancy and no special precautions are required. Any limitations relate to the underlying cardiac disorder.

Surgery. The major risk, although small, during surgery pertains to the use of diathermy, both cutting and cauterizing. Modern pacemakers use bipolar leads (see above) and although it is difficult to interfere with the sensing of the pacemaker, diathermy should be kept at least 10 cm away from the pacing generator and ECG recording should be carried out throughout. If close diathermy cannot be avoided, the pacemaker can be protected by placing a strong magnet over the pacing can. This temporarily turns off the sensing circuits and allows the pacemaker to pace continuously. The magnet can be applied during the course of the surgery. The pacemaker reverts to its normal function as soon as the magnet is withdrawn.

MRI scanning. A recent development is MRI-safe pacemakers. Unless the device is specifically designed to be MRI safe, no pacemaker or defibrillator is safe inside an MRI scanner. MRI scanning can still be performed if necessary but great care and close monitoring is required.

Transcutaneous electrical nerve stimulators should not be used close to a pacing generator.

Daily activities. Pacemakers confer very few restrictions on daily activity. Normal sexual function and exercise is allowed and depends purely on the underlying cardiac abnormality. Strenuous exertion such as swimming is best avoided for 1 month. Wearers may use microwave ovens but should not stand too close.

Mobile/cellular phones can interfere with pacemaker function and it is recommended that the phone be used in the ear opposite to the pacemaker.

Implantable cardioverter defibrillators

Indications. Implantable cardioverter defibrillators (ICDs) are the treatment of choice for patients with life-threatening ventricular tachycardias. ICDs monitor heart rhythm and shock the heart if there is a rhythm problem. All ICDs have back-up pacemakers that prevent the heart from slowing down too much after the shock is delivered.

Primary prevention. Many patients die suddenly, often out of hospital, as a result of hemodynamically unstable ventricular tachycardia (VT) or ventricular fibrillation (VF) in the context of ischemic heart disease or impaired LV function. The ability to better predict such an outcome has enabled cardiologists to focus on prevention of these sudden deaths. An ICD is capable of detecting a fast heart rhythm and automatically delivers a cardioverting shock. It is a life-saving device. Indications for use of ICDs as a primary preventive measure are shown in Table 11.2. The primary prevention trials MADIT and MUSTT showed that patients with ICDs had more than a 50% survival benefit compared with control groups, despite the use of amiodarone in 75% of control patients in the MADIT trial. The MADIT-II trial, which randomized 1232 patients with any history of a remote myocardial infarction (MI) and LV dysfunction (ejection fraction < 30–35%) to receive an ICD or to continue medical therapy, showed a 31% reduction in the risk of death after ICD implantation. Although good news clinically, the results raise difficult questions about the potentially crippling economic impact of this added

TABLE 11.2

Indications for primary prevention with an ICD

- Depressed left ventricular systolic function (ejection fraction ≤ 35%)
- Cardiac conditions with a high risk of sudden death
  - Long-QT syndrome
  - Hypertrophic cardiomyopathy
  - Brugada syndrome
  - Arrhythmogenic right ventricular dysplasia
  - After repair of tetralogy of Fallot

healthcare cost. Many studies have shown that LV systolic function is the main predictor of sudden death.

Secondary prevention includes patients who have survived an out-of-hospital cardiac arrest or who have symptomatic sustained VT. A meta-analysis of secondary prevention studies has shown a 28% reduction in the relative risk of death with the ICD, which is almost entirely due to a 50% reduction in the risk of sudden death.

Heart failure. Many patients who are at risk of sudden death have poor LV function. In some cases, the addition of a third pacing lead in the coronary sinus veins allows LV pacing and resynchronization of ventricular contraction (see pages 128–30). As patients who are eligible for CRT have poor ventricular function and are at high risk of sudden death, many CRT devices also have defibrillators (CRT-D). These devices improve symptoms by their biventricular effects and reduce sudden death by defibrillation.

Implantation. ICDs are implanted either subcutaneously, as for a pacemaker, in the left or right deltopectoral area, or (rarely) submuscularly in thin patients to avoid future device erosion. The ventricular lead tip can be positioned in the RVA or the right ventricular outflow tract (RVOT); a second lead can be positioned in the right atrial appendage to allow DDD pacing, if required, and discrimination between atrial and ventricular tachycardias. The ventricular defibrillator lead has either one or two shocking coils. For two-coil leads, one is proximal (usually within the superior vena cava) and one is distal (right ventricle). Implantation is associated with mortality of approximately 0.1%.

Testing. The unit is tested during implantation with the patient still under conscious sedation. VF is induced and an intracardiac shock given to determine that the VF is correctly sensed and that enough shock energy was given to defibrillate successfully. Satisfactory sensing during sinus rhythm, VT and VF, as well as pacing and defibrillatory thresholds, are established. Defibrillatory thresholds should be at least 10 J less than the maximum output of the defibrillator (approximately 36 J). Biphasic shocks are more effective than monophasic shocks.

Complications

Short-term complications are essentially the same as for pacemakers and include infection and lead problems (see page 131).

Long-term complications are related to inappropriate shocks for sinus tachycardia or atrial arrhythmias, which can be particularly problematic because patients are often awake and shocks are painful. Patients describe it as: 'like being kicked in the chest by a horse'.

Many patients with ICDs also take concomitant antiarrhythmic therapy, which helps to reduce potential ICD usage.

Product recalls warrant closer monitoring of the patient (see pages 142–3).

ICD function

Mode of action. An ICD consists of a battery, one or two leads inserted into the heart, a capacitor to deliver the charge and a detection algorithm capable of determining VF and VT. The shock delivery lead is positioned in the right ventricle and constantly senses the underlying heart rate. The device can determine the onset of tachycardia and delivers pre-programmed therapies that are set by the implanting physician and are often patient specific. If the heart rate is very fast, it is assumed the rhythm is VF and a defibrillating shock is given. If the rhythm is relatively slow it may be possible to terminate the arrhythmia by using pacing protocols (see below). However, if there is any doubt, a shock is given.

Pacing therapy for tachycardia control, if successful, is painless and avoids a potentially painful shock. In slower tachycardias the patient may be conscious and may receive a painful shock. As previously mentioned, all ICDs have back-up pacemakers within the generator.

Pace termination of ventricular tachycardias. Both supraventricular tachycardia (SVT) and VT can be terminated by pacing techniques, although the advent of curative therapy in the form of radiofrequency ablation (RFA) has made pace termination obsolete for SVTs (see Chapter 6). In many cases, VT responds to termination by pacing in the ventricle. There are two methods of pace termination: underdrive (no longer used routinely) and overdrive pacing.

Overdrive pacing is effective, painless and quick, and is associated with low battery drain. The device detects a change in heart rate and applies a short sequence of rapid anti-tachycardia pacing (ATP). Sometimes rapid pacing in the ventricle can induce VF or accelerate a VT (possibly converting it from a stable to an unstable arrhythmia), so all devices able to terminate VT must have defibrillatory capability (Figure 11.9). VT is an important re-entrant arrhythmia in ischemic heart disease and, in many instances, can be treated effectively by overdrive pacing.

ICD developments. An important development is the ICD's ability to record intracardiac signals (electrograms), which allows monitoring of each episode of ATP or defibrillation. If therapy has been inappropriate, then the programming can be changed using a programming unit placed over the ICD site. Current ICDs employ ATP with the availability of low- and higher-energy shocks – tiered therapy. ATP can take the form of adaptive burst pacing, with a cycle length of 80–90% of that of the VT. Pacing bursts can be fixed (constant cycle length) or autodecremental (ramp pacing) where the pacing burst accelerates (each cycle becomes faster as the pacing train progresses). Should ATP fail, low-energy shocks are given first to try to terminate VT with the minimum of pain (as some patients remain conscious despite rapid VT).

With the advent of dual-chamber systems and improved diagnostic algorithms, shocking is mostly avoided during atrial arrhythmias. Even in single-lead systems, the algorithms are now sufficiently sophisticated to differentiate between most atrial arrhythmias and VT on the basis of the tachycardia characteristics such as sudden onset, rate stability and QRS width. The rate stability function assesses the cycle length and variability, which helps to exclude AF. However, inappropriate shock delivery during AF is still the most common complication related to ICDs and may occur in up to 30% of cases.

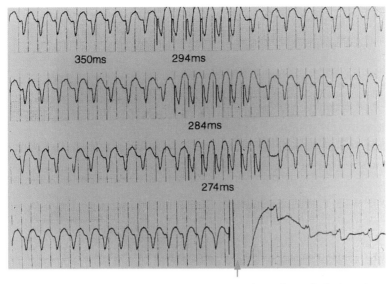

350ms   294ms

284ms

274ms

Figure 11.9 Anti-tachycardia pacing during ventricular tachycardia (VT). VT is present at the start of the strip. The device detects the change in heart rate and applies a short sequence of rapid paced beats. VT is not terminated, so the device reapplies a further two episodes of paced beats, both of which it correctly determines have been ineffective. As a result, the device applies a small (1 Joule) intracardiac shock (arrow) which terminates the VT to sinus rhythm.

Effect on quality of life

Psychological issues. The implantation of an ICD is a major decision. The ICD constantly reminds patients they have a life-threatening condition and although many patients are reassured by the technology, in some the device can induce severe anxiety. Patients may occasionally undergo psychological counseling before implantation, and some may require further counseling afterwards. One of the most debilitating events is the inappropriate intracardiac shock delivery, which may provoke anxiety that requires treatment.

Driving. As for pacemakers, regulations for return to driving after implantation of an ICD vary between countries (and between States in the USA). In general, commercial driving is prohibited and personal driving is prohibited for 6 months following implantation of a defibrillator where there have been symptoms associated with the arrhythmia. In the UK, if a shock is delivered within this period, the license is withheld for a further

141

6 months. Any change in therapy programming or in antiarrhythmic medication means a month of abstinence, and all patients must be reviewed regularly. Patients are prohibited indefinitely if they experience incapacity with no diagnosis, or for 4 weeks if it is controlled to the satisfaction of the cardiologist.

Removal of pacemakers and defibrillators

The presence of infection mandates removal of all parts of the system, leads and generator. Lead extraction is a challenge and carries a small but significant risk. There are two methods: open-heart surgery, a procedure with a 1% mortality and a moderate morbidity, or percutaneous lead extraction, which involves the use of a cutting device (e.g. either cutting sheaths or a laser or radiofrequency cutter) to remove the leads from the heart. Leads become fibrosed at certain points in the heart, classically at the lead/myocardium interface and at the junction of the superior vena cava and the right atrium. Tearing of the great vein or the right ventricle is a recognized complication with catastrophic results. The overall mortality associated with percutaneous lead extraction is 1–3%. Lead extraction should be the last resort and patients must be counseled accordingly. Whether removal is by the percutaneous route or via open-heart surgery is a clinical decision and should take into account the patient's choice.

Pacemakers and ICDs must be removed before cremation because of the risk of explosion during incineration. ICDs that are temporarily disabled and removed must be packaged and labeled appropriately to prevent accidental shock to personnel.

Device failures and recalls

Regular checks (annually for a pacemaker and usually 6-monthly for an ICD) will nearly always identify any early failures and premature battery depletion. In addition, some devices can self test and provide a vibration alarm or a beep through the device if there is a problem. While manufacturing faults with generator components are now rare, leads remain an engineering challenge. In recent years there have been two major worldwide recalls involving a defibrillation lead (by separate manufacturers). All patients with these leads have required regular and frequent surveillance and, in some cases, the leads have had to be extracted. Although most systems are highly reliable, regular follow up is mandatory in order to detect any future faults. Device revision or explant carries small but significant risks, and the benefits and risks must be discussed with each patient on an individual basis.

Remote monitoring

The majority of current devices have the capability of transmitting information wirelessly to either a mobile phone-based system or via a telemetry wand to a land-based phone line. The data can then be monitored remotely while the patient is at home. This is ideal for rural areas and it is hoped that repeat visits to the pacing clinics may become obsolete. Information can be sent on a daily basis giving a detailed picture of the device. Heart failure monitoring, with the patients at home, is being intensively investigated to predict if an acute decompensation is imminent and prevent hospital readmission. Currently, interrogation is unidirectional. Due to safety concerns devices cannot be reprogrammed at a distance.

Future trends

Developing technologies are extending the indications for pacemaker implantation. Leadless pacemakers are being developed. A leadless defibrillator is already available and has proven successful in early clinical trials. Advances in genetic engineering may allow cellular pacemakers that can restimulate dormant cardiac cells and in 20 years time these may replace conventional battery-based pacemakers.

Key points – cardiac devices: pacemakers and defibrillators

- Pacemakers are the treatment of choice in patients with symptomatic bradycardia.
- All implantable defibrillators have a back-up pacemaker.
- Patients with pacemakers can live a near-normal life.
- Patients need regular review (usually annually) to check battery life and lead integrity.

Key references

Adán V, Crown LA. Diagnosis and treatment of sick sinus syndrome. *Am Fam Physician* 2003;67:1725–32.

Buch E, Boyle NG, Belott PH. Pacemaker and defibrillator lead extraction. *Circulation* 2011;123: e378–80.

Cleland JG, Daubert JC, Erdmann E et al.; CARE-HF Study Investigators. The effect of cardiac resynchronization on morbidity and mortality in heart failure. *N Engl J Med* 2005;352: 1539–49.

Cubbon RM, Witte KK. Cardiac resynchronisation therapy for chronic heart failure and conduction delay. *BMJ* 2009;338:b1265.

Daubert JC, Saxon L, Adamson PB et al. 2012 EHRA/HRS expert consensus statement on cardiac resynchronization therapy in heart failure: implant and follow-up recommendations and management. *Heart Rhythm* 2012;9:1524–76.

ESC. Guidelines for cardiac pacing and cardiac resynchronization therapy: The Task Force for Cardiac Pacing and Cardiac Resynchronization Therapy of the European Society of Cardiology. *Eur Heart J* 2007;28:2256–95.

ESC. 2010 ESC guidelines on device therapy in HF: 3. cardiac resynchronization therapy with defibrillator function in patients with heart failure in New York Heart Association function class I/II. *Europace* 2010;12:1526–36.

Heart Rhythm Society. Transvenous Lead Extraction: Heart Rhythm Society Expert Consensus on Facilities, Training, Indications, and Patient Management, 2009. www.HRSonline. org/Policy/ClinicalGuidelines

Mangrum JM, DiMarco JP. The evaluation and management of bradycardia. *N Engl J Med* 2000;342:703–9.

Michaelsson M, Engle MA. Congenital complete heart block: an international study of the natural history. *Cardiovasc Clin* 1972;4:85–101.

Odemuyiwa O, Camm AJ. Prophylactic pacing for prevention of sudden death in congenital heart block. *Pacing Clin Electrophysiol* 1992;15:1526–30.

Toff WD, Camm AJ, Skehan JD; United Kingdom Pacing and Cardiovascular Events Trial Investigators. Single-chamber versus dual-chamber pacing for high-grade atrioventricular shock. *N Engl J Med* 2005;353:145–55.

Van Eck JW, van Hemel NM, Zuithof P et al. Incidence and predictors of in-hospital events after first implantation of pacemakers. *Europace* 2007;9:884–9.

Yerra L, Reddy PC. Effects of electromagnetic interference on implanted cardiac devices and their management. *Cardiol Rev* 2007;15:304–9.

Useful resources

UK
Anticoagulation Europe
www.anticoagulationeurope.org

Arrhythmia Alliance
www.heartrhythmcharity.org.uk
Defibs saves lives campaign:
www.defibssavelives.org

Atrial Fibrillation Association
www.atrialfibrillation.org.uk

British Cardiovascular Society
www.bcs.com

British Heart Rhythm Society
www.bhrs.com

USA
American College of Cardiology
www.acc.org

American Heart Association
www.heart.org/HEARTORG

Heart Rhythm Society
www.hrsonline.org

StopAfib.org
www.stopafib.org

International
Canadian Heart Rhythm Society
www.chrsonline.ca

European Society of Cardiology
www.escardio.org

Heart Foundation (Australia)
www.heartfoundation.org.au

Further reading
Bonow RO, Mann DL, Zipes DP, Libby P, eds. *Braunwald's Heart Disease: A Textbook of Cardiovascular Medicine*, 9th edn. Saunders, 2011.

Ellenbogen KA, Wood MA, eds. *Cardiac Pacing and ICDs*, 5th edn. Wiley-Blackwell, 2008.

Hayes DL, Wang PJ, Sackner-Bernstein J, Asirvatham SJ. *Resynchronization and Defibrillation for Heart Failure: A Practical Approach*. Wiley-Blackwell, 2004.

Josephson ME. *Clinical Cardiac Electrophysiology: Techniques and Interpretations*, 4th edn. Lippincott Williams & Wilkins, 2008.

Zipes D, Haissaguerre M, eds. *Catheter Ablation of Arrythmias*, 2nd edn. Wiley-Blackwell, 2002.

Zipes DP, Jalife J, eds. *Cardiac Electrophysiology: From Cell to Bedside*, 5th edn. Philadelphia: Saunders, 2009.

Index

147